Youthful, glowing skin can be yours with: THE ACNE CURE

"Dr. Dubrow has come up with a wonderful program to treat acne."
—Robert Schwartz, M.D., plastic surgeon certified by
the American Board of Plastic Surgery, Dallas

"A wonderful program based on sound medical science."
—Harry G. Preuss, M.D., F.A.C.N., C.N.S., professor of medicine
and pathology, Georgetown University Medical Center, Washington,
D.C., and author of *The Prostate Cure* and *Maitaka Magic*

"An excellent tome for patients and physicians alike."
—Malcom A. Lesavoy, M.D., F.A.C.S., clinical professor, division of
plastic and reconstructive surgery, UCLA School of Medicine,
and plastic surgeon certified by the American
Board of Plastic Surgery, Los Angeles

"THE ACNE CURE provides a sound, logical approach to treating acne."
—Kenny R. Mallott, M.D., dermatologist certified by the
American Board of Dermatology, Kihei, Hawaii

"We've been using this system in our practice for a considerable
time, with wonderful results."
—Peter Helton, D.O., dermatologist certified by the American
Osteopathic Board of Dermatology, Newport Beach, California

"I recommend this book to all my patients suffering from acne."
—Randall D. Haworth, M.D., plastic surgeon certified by the
American Board of Plastic Surgery, Beverly Hills, California

THE
ACNE
CURE

THE NONPRESCRIPTION PLAN
THAT SHOWS DRAMATIC RESULTS
IN AS LITTLE AS 24 HOURS

TERRY J. DUBROW, M.D.
AND BRENDA D. ADDERLY, M.H.A.

WARNER BOOKS

NEW YORK   BOSTON

This work is dedicated to my loving wife, Heather Paige Kent,
who continues to inspire, amaze, and amuse me every day of my life.
—Terry J. Dubrow, M.D.

For Peter, Connor and Evan's daddy.
—Brenda D. Adderly, M.H.A.

NOTICE: The information herein is not intended to be a substitute for medical advice. You are advised to consult with your health care professional with regard to matters relating to your health, and in particular regarding matters that may require diagnosis or medical attention.

Mention of specific companies, organizations, or authorities in this book does not imply endorsement by the publisher, nor does mention of specific companies, organizations, or authorities imply that they endorse this book.

Internet addresses and telephone numbers given in this book were accurate at the time it went to press.

Warner Books Edition

Copyright © 2003 by Terry J. Dubrow, M.D., and Brenda D. Adderly, M.H.A.
All rights reserved.

This Warner Books edition is published by arrangement with Rodale, 33 East Minor Street, Emmaus, PA 18089-0099.

Warner Books

Time Warner Book Group
1271 Avenue of the Americas, New York, NY 10020
Visit our Web site at www.twbookmark.com

Printed in the United States of America

First Warner Books Printing: May 2004

10 9 8 7 6 5 4 3

The Library of Congress has cataloged the hardcover edition as follows:
Dubrow, Terry J.
     The acne cure : the revolutionary nonprescription treatment plan that
cures even the most severe acne and shows dramatic results in as little as
24 hours / Terry J. Dubrow and Brenda D. Adderly.
          p.   cm.
     Includes bibliographical references and index.
     ISBN 1-57954-742-7 hardcover
     1. Acne—Popular works.   I. Adderly, Brenda.   II. Title.
RL131.D83   2003
616.5'3—dc21   2002156617

ISBN: 0-446-69241-7 (pbk.)

CONTENTS

ACKNOWLEDGMENTS

THREE PEOPLE HAVE BEEN OF GREAT HELP TO US in the preparation of this book, and we want to thank them most sincerely. . .

Howard Cohl, president of MI-5, and a longtime friend, conceived of this project and wrote the draft of the original proposal. Without him, there would be no book.

Peter Engel, Brenda Adderly's husband, took time off from his own writing projects to provide a lot of useful help in the writing of this book.

And Jeremy Katz, our editor at Rodale, has once again proven that he is one of the most intelligent, practical, and effective editors in publishing.

1

SKIN

DR. TERRY DUBROW'S WIFE, HEATHER PAIGE KENT, star of the CBS drama *That's Life*, awoke one morning, appalled. "Terry, look at my face! I've totally broken out. I'm due on the set in three days. Is there anything you can do?"

Of course, Heather knew that her husband, a board-certified plastic surgeon and director of the Acne Clinic of Newport Beach, California, had been working on protocols to cure acne quickly and safely. What she didn't yet know was that he had finally found the answer. The panic she felt was based on her assumption that acne is only partially treatable, if at all.

That assumption is false. This is the truth:

Using the techniques outlined in this book,
acne can be completely eliminated in
95 percent of all cases—even the most severe
ones—in 6 weeks or less. These techniques start
to work in 24 hours.

In the remaining 5 percent of the cases, the Acne Cure program will generally reduce the severity of acne. Later in the book, we will discuss what additional steps you can take to get rid of the remaining traces of the disease—even in the toughest cases.

Whether you're White, Black, Asian, or Hispanic; whether you're a teenage boy with pimples or a mature man suffering from acne aggravated by razor bumps and ingrown beard hairs; whether you're a teenage girl who feels she can't get a date because of her zits, or a woman whose face is disfigured by the blotchy inflammation of severe acne, your condition can be cured.

When we say "cured," we mean that in almost all cases—even the toughest—the acne cure program we describe in this book will eliminate virtually all blemishes, inflammation, redness, whiteheads, and blackheads within no more than 6 weeks. Milder cases may be resolved in only a few days or even—as in Heather's case—overnight. Sure, there may be recurrences (although they are unlikely if you stick to the maintenance program), but they too can be rapidly resolved, usually in just a few days.

And if that isn't a cure, we don't know what is!

Some purists argue that getting rid of the symptoms but knowing that in some cases they may return means that this is not a full cure. All we know is that, like hundreds of Dr. Dubrow's other patients, male and female, Heather's acne disappeared. Three days after her skin eruptions, Heather went back to work with a smile on her face, and not a blemish in sight.

In the next few chapters, we will describe exactly how the cure works. However, first you have to understand what skin is, how it works, and what you can do to keep it healthy throughout your life. Not only is healthy skin less likely to be attacked by acne or other skin diseases, but it also looks so much better.

And who doesn't want young-looking, healthy, glowing acne-free skin?

WHAT DOES SKIN DO?

Simply stated, skin is a miracle. We think you'll agree by the end of this chapter.

Just consider some of your skin's extraordinary qualities:

• **Treated properly, it stays with you—and in good working condition—for a lifetime.** No manmade flexible protective covering lasts nearly that long. Plastic becomes stiff and cracks. Rubber degenerates. Of course, if you continue to abuse your skin month after month, year after year, you will eventually harm it so that it too will start to show its age. Even so, it will never stop working. You may succumb to the breakdown of your circulatory system. You may even suffer from skin cancer that can metastasize elsewhere in your body and prove lethal. You may succumb to heart failure. But you are unlikely to die of skin failure!

• **It repairs itself.** When you scratch leather, it stays scratched; when you cut it, the cut remains forever. But before it was leather, it was living animal skin. It repaired—and healed—its scratches quickly, efficiently, and generally without a trace. And it repaired even the deepest gash with only a surface scar remaining. Your skin works in the same remarkable way.

• **It is wonderfully elastic and pliable.** At any moment, your skin can stretch and contract as well as an elastic band; we call this *immediate elasticity*. Also, a woman's abdomen expands during pregnancy to several times its original size and then contracts to the way it was; we call that *long-term elasticity*. Moreover, at each stage of that long-term elasticity, your skin also maintains its immediate elasticity. Remarkable!

If you ever watch a heavyweight boxing match, you cannot help but marvel at how the fighters' skin can withstand such vicious blows. Yet, although the skin may bruise or be cut, it never breaks down. It is sensitive enough to feel the touch of a feather, or the lightest kiss, yet tough enough to withstand the most violent abuse.

• **It registers sensations with such specificity that it lets the brain differentiate among them.** Thus, we can tell instantly whether our skin is being pricked by a needle or scratched by a rose, whether the water is cold or warm or hot, and whether a peach is smooth and velvety ripe, or wrinkled and too soft to eat. Even when we are asleep, our sense of touch keeps working: If a fly lands on your nose, you will swipe it away and stay asleep; if you develop an itch, you will scratch it without waking yourself.

• **It not only feels but also remembers sensations.** If you have been lying for too long on one patch of skin (so that a pressure sore becomes a risk) your skin's ability to feel the pressure, remember its duration, and transmit that information to your brain will cause you to turn in your sleep.

• **It is incredibly resilient.** Through its regenerative qualities, your skin withstands ultraviolet light strong enough to fade drapes in months, acid rain that can erode cathedral stones, and a constant round of burns, bangs, abrasions, and bruises that would leave most manmade materials threadbare and riddled with holes.

• **It routinely changes color to help withstand sun damage.** If you are exposed to increasing sun gradually (which would apply to prehistoric man as spring turned to summer), your skin adapts by giving you a tan and, so, avoids the pain of sunburn. Of course, if you suddenly expose your winter skin to intense sunlight (say, by flying to Florida on vacation), your skin cannot adapt fast enough because it did not evolve for that eventuality. We should add, however, that even though your tan protects your skin against immediate sunburn, no skin—not even the darkest African-American skin—is immune to long-term damage from ultraviolet light.

• **It has a built-in cooling mechanism.** When your body overheats, your skin comes to the rescue. If your skin didn't sweat—and the sweat evaporate to cool you down—your whole biological system would break down in hot weather.

• **It is largely self-cleaning and rarely suffers from lasting infections.** The skin continually replenishes its healthy layer of sebum— a slightly acidic mixture of oil, water, enzymes, and various bacteria fighters. In doing so, it keep itself clean and largely infection-free in two ways.

One is that it physically dislodges most of the dirt and detritus that would otherwise encrust your skin. This cleaning function, which was far more important before we had widespread running water and other cleaning facilities, is remarkably efficient. If you examine the body of someone who has worked all day in a dusty atmosphere, you will see that, apart from their hands (or other areas) that were directly exposed to the dirt, the skin is remarkably dirt-free.

As many of you know, when you get an itch in the middle of your back, your arms just can't reach to scratch it. This applies especially to men (and to many of us as we age) because our shoulders and arms tend to be less flexible. Of course, that means you cannot reach there to wash, either. Yet that patch of unreachable skin, treated only with clear water from the shower or bath, is no dirtier than the adjacent skin that has been washed with soap.

The other advantage of the sebum is that, although skin is prone to attack 24 hours a day by any number of germs, viruses, insects, and fungi, sebum is fungi- and bacterio-static, so the skin rarely succumbs to infections. And even when it does, in most cases they go away pretty quickly. (That, of course, is why acne can be such a curse. Untreated, it is one of the worst things that ever happens to most people's skin.)

• **It can let in certain important elements even while protecting you from others.** It does a superb job of keeping out water that would soak through most rain garments. That's why you can swim without becoming waterlogged. But it can let in a certain amount of oxygen needed for the skin to "breathe," and it can absorb enough water vapor to keep itself moist in most conditions. It can even let in certain chemicals, such as medicines. That is why nicotine patches work.

• **Most astonishing of all, our skin is capable of holding in the entire, huge amount of liquid that flows through our bodies.** When your doctor tells you that your blood pressure is a healthy 120 over 80, he is talking about a lot of pressure! Just think how the blood pours out of even a small cut on your forehead or how a crack in the skin inside your nose causes the blood to stream out, and you can imagine how much internal pressure the skin is able to withstand—and all without your even noticing!

As you consider this list of skin's amazing properties, it becomes obvious that it must be a vastly complex organ. Indeed it is.

WHAT IS SKIN?

Most descriptions of skin explain that it consists of three layers: the epidermis, which is the outer layer; the dermis, which is the main part of the skin; and the subcutaneous, or fatty layer at the base of the skin. However, while correct, this oversimplification clouds rather than enlightens our understanding of skin.

For one thing, layering implies a fairly uniform formation of skin wherever it is found. In fact, there are huge differences: the skin on your eyelids is paper thin. It consists mostly of highly flexible material, and it has relatively little "horny" outer protection. On the other hand, the skin on the sole of your foot is 5 millimeters (about $1/8$ inch) thick, mostly consisting of inelastic, "horny" material. But even this is not uniform. Skin thickness varies among people depending on what use they make of the skin on various parts of their bodies.

For example, if you (or your kids) go barefoot around the yard when it gets warm in the summer, you'll soon see the skin on your feet thicken to protect you against damage. And no doubt Indian fakirs who have learned to walk on hot coals have developed skin on the soles of their feet that is a great deal thicker than yours!

To fully understand how skin works, we should consider the many separate functions it fulfills and see how each of its layers and other component parts allows it to fulfill each of those functions.

HOW DOES SKIN FUNCTION?

Our skin protects us—and continues to do so year after year throughout our lives—because it replaces itself constantly. In young people, the entire skin is replaced within less than a month. In old folks, it may take the body as long as 45 days to replace the skin. During an 80-year lifetime, then, we do not live in a single skin but in almost 1,000 different skins. (Snakes shed their skin as they grow. But they do so episodically; we do the same thing constantly.)

This regenerative process has the obvious advantage of replacing any damaged, discolored, or otherwise shopworn skin with new skin. However, it has a second huge advantage, namely that the dead skin cells—now dry and as hard and horny as your nails—form a barrier called the stratum corneum. Although this layer is quite thin, it holds back most of your skin's attackers. It does so most effectively where the skin is under the greatest attack, accommodating itself accordingly—hence the tough, calloused skin on the hands of manual laborers, as compared with the soft surface on the hands of a typical computer techie.

The Stratum Corneum

The stratum corneum (Latin for "horny layer") consists of dead skin cells that, in losing their living nuclei as they are pushed to the surface by new cells forming underneath them, have been flattened into tiny flakes. These flakes, by their shape, interlock into a shielding veneer.

In young skin, this veneer layer is rapidly replaced by new cells and therefore accounts for a smaller proportion of the skin's thickness. Consequently, the color of the living skin can "glow" through better. Also, since the stratum corneum of young skin is subjected to a shorter period of wear and tear (as it is more rapidly replaced), it is smoother than the same layer in older skin. In combination, this smooth glow is what we define as a youthful complexion.

In older skin, while the stratum corneum may be thinner (since it is not replaced as rapidly by new cells), since it also sloughs off less rapidly, it nevertheless represents a higher proportion of the whole skin. The effect is that there is less inner "glow" and that what there is tends to be masked. Or, as one elderly lady told us acerbically, "Honey, I haven't blushed in years!" In addition, because it remains in place longer, the stratum corneum of older skin tends to have what amount to tiny erosions, which, both to the touch and to the naked eye, appear as grayish, rough, dry skin. Less glow and a rough surface is what we describe as a tired or aging complexion.

The Epidermis

Immediately under the stratum corneum (which is actually the dead portion of the epidermis) is the living portion of the epidermis. This consists of many layers of cells, called keratinocytes, that generate keratin, the tough protein that represents about 95 percent of what we call our skin. The keratinocytes form at the bottom of the epidermis as tiny round cells, then shuffle their way to the surface, becoming flatter as they progress, until—flat dead, so to speak—they become the bottom of the stratum corneum.

The epidermis also contains another important type of cells, called melanocytes. These produce the melanin that darkens our skin to try to protect it from damaging ultraviolet light. Surprisingly, all skin contains the same number of melanocytes. The skin's color is determined not by how many melanocytes we have but by the number, size, and color of the melanin pigment granules each melanocyte produces. Thus, a person with darker skin has melanocytes that produce more, larger, and darker pigment "granules" than a person with lighter skin.

Actually, melanocytes are very clever cells. When we view them under a microscope after they've been exposed to sun, it looks as if the darkened melanin cells have deposited themselves on top of the skin's DNA-containing skin cells, almost as if they were trying to shield those nuclei from damage. Only when the melanocytes are overexerted in the extreme—such as from excess sun exposure or some other external damaging impact—do they sometimes go awry and develop melanoma, a particularly vicious form of skin cancer.

Finally, the epidermis also contains Langerhans cells. It's believed that these specialized cells provide a warning to the body's immune system to prepare to fight some external damaging material, such as the toxins from poison ivy or poison oak.

The Dermis

The epidermis, although very strong, is only a thin layer and therefore has only limited resistance. However, under it, providing strength and support, is the solid portion of our skin, called the dermis. The dermis, which consists primarily of collagen and elastin, is where most of the action of our skin takes place.

Collagen is the main protein that constitutes skin (also our ligaments and tendons). It consists of fibroblasts, tiny submarine-shaped cells that produce spiral chains of collagen molecules. The collagen chains join to form braids of collagen, which are woven into bundles that form into netlike structures that represent some 70 percent of the dermis. These collagen "nets," which under a microscope look rather like a loose pile of twigs, provide our skin with its remarkable strength and durability.

The other vital dermis constituent is elastin—filaments of protein that are, indeed, highly elastic. When stretched, the elastin causes the skin to snap back to its previous shape. Unfortunately, as a result of sun exposure, smoking, and other insults, elastin loses its elasticity, causing older skin to sag, rather than snap back.

Despite innumerable claims to the contrary, you can't replace collagen or elastin by taking pills or applying creams that contain those substances. Pills don't work because they are digested in the stomach and never reach their destination. The creams don't work because both collagen and elastin molecules are too large to penetrate the stratum corneum and the epidermis to reach the dermis. Indeed, as we shall discuss later, the only way to increase collagen is to use Retin-A (chemically, tretinoin, a vitamin A–type compound).

Retin-A, a prescription drug, is not the same as Retinol or other vitamin A chemicals sold as ingredients in over-the-counter "anti-aging" creams. Even Retin-A cannot add collagen to your skin. Retin-A does, however, induce the skin to produce more collagen. The product must be used with a certain amount of caution because it strips the stratum corneum and, to some extent, even the epidermis. For some people, Retin-A may do more harm than good.

COSMETIC ADVERTISING EXAGGERATES

While you probably don't believe everything you read or hear in cosmetic ads (or other ads, for that matter), you may ask how cosmetic companies can make skin-rejuvenating claims for products that don't rejuvenate the skin. Doesn't that contravene truth-in-advertising laws?

The answer lies in the clever wording the cosmetic companies use in their advertising. They say, "makes your skin *look* younger" (or similar words) rather than "makes your skin younger." Technically, any cream, oil, or fat will temporarily make your skin "look" younger. Coating skin in that way blocks a certain amount of its moisture from evaporating. That slightly plumped-up look does indeed seem more youthful—for a short time.

Another clever type of wording used to advertise certain creams is along the lines of "helps preserve your skin from aging." If the cream contains a sunblock, this is a true claim. Anything you do to reduce the amount of ultraviolet light hitting your skin will slow down the aging process.

Finally, as we shall discuss in detail later, antioxidants can fight off many of the damaging effects of ultraviolet light and various types of pollution by combining with the damaging free oxygen radicals that are caused by these insults. Thus, creams that contain effective antioxidants may also slow down (or even help to repair) skin damage, and thus the appearance of aging. However, all the other additives mentioned in the same ad, although they may smell nice or feel silky on your skin, do little else but just that: smell nice and feel silky.

Unfortunately, so far no collagen or elastin replacement cream has been invented. Of course, new skin care products are introduced almost daily. Thus, it is possible that before long science will find a way to regenerate collagen and/or elastin. However, until such a product or methodology is discovered, we suggest that you read the cosmetic ads with great care to find their hidden meanings—and then take them with not just a pinch but a whole bucket of salt!

HOW SKIN AGES

Since skin renews itself every 28 to 45 days, how is it that old skin shows its age?

Partly, as stated above, that is because, as we age and new skin cells form less rapidly, the stratum corneum becomes a larger percentage of our skin, thus seeming more opaque and feeling rougher. However, the main reason that our skin "shows its age" is that, when we damage its basic structure, even though the epidermis will completely regenerate itself without scars, the dermis will not. It just cannot completely recover from the damage we do. Indeed, any time you cut into the dermis, you are bound to create some scar, however small.

The smaller and "cleaner" the damage to your skin (that is, neatly cut rather than ripped and with jagged edges), the smaller will be the scar. But some scarring will always remain, though it may not be visible to the naked eye. Now, over time, even if you do not cut the skin with a knife or scrape it off in a bicycle or car accident, you damage it day in and day out with ultraviolet light. This light breaks down the elastin molecules in the dermis so that, under a microscope, instead of looking like a web of long strands, they look like piles of short sticks. With a reduced amount of healthy elastin, the skin is less capable of snapping back into place. As a result, like the surface of a badly made bed, creases and wrinkles appear.

These wrinkles are then exacerbated by an aging phenomenon that has nothing to do with the skin itself but rather with the muscles beneath it. They become weaker and looser and therefore sag, causing the skin over them to be pulled out of shape. To accommodate a "sag," your skin stretches. Elsewhere, the excess skin, no longer as elastic as it used to be, doesn't fully retract. The overall effect is that your skin literally no longer exactly fits your face and, like a slipcover on a sofa whose springs have collapsed, any number of unsightly wrinkles result.

This explanation, of course, begs the question why do our muscles sag. To answer this, we must first explain just how the muscles work in the first place.

When you want to move a muscle in your face—say, to smile or frown—your brain sends an electric signal through a series of nerves that activate the muscle in question. But the nerves do not connect directly to the muscle. Rather, each nerve ends in a small, bulblike vessel adjacent to the muscle that contains two chemicals: acetylcholine and dimethylyaminoethanol. The electrical signal from the brain causes the nerve endings to release these chemicals, which cause the muscles to contract.

As we age, the body produces less of these chemicals, and therefore the muscles become looser, with less ability to contract. In short, they sag.

Of course, we are still not at the base of the answer, for the final question remains, Why do our bodies produce less of many desirable chemicals, including acetylcholine, and how do outside factors such as ultraviolet light and smoking create this damaging effect?

The answer is complicated and perhaps not yet fully understood by medical science. However, there is no doubt that one major cause of these problems is the formation of so-called free radicals.

Free Radicals

In essence, free radicals are oxygen molecules that, in the course of many of our normal bodily functions, such as breathing or digesting our food, have lost an electron. They are therefore unstable until they can combine with an electron, which they must "steal" from a complete molecule in the vicinity. Usually, this system is pretty much in balance, with the number of free radicals kept in a stable proportion to the number of whole molecules. However, the presence of certain outside factors—such as long-term exposure to sunlight, cigarette smoke, or various pollutants—increases the percentage of free radicals in the system. Under those circumstances, the free radicals can break down the skin's elastin and cause premature sagging and thus the appearance of aging.

Scientists have long known about free radicals and have indicted them as a contributory cause of any number of diseases. However, the science surrounding how they work and the damage they can do is still relatively incomplete.

We do know that free radicals seem to attack every part of the human cell: the nucleus, where DNA, our bodies' key building block, is generated; the fats (lipids) that reside inside our cells; and the cell membrane, which constitutes the outer layer of our cells. However, there remains scientific controversy as to whether the aging effect we see throughout our bodies, and of course on our skin, is primarily a result of damage to the cells' nuclei—and thus to the DNA being generated there—or of damage to the outer layer of the skin, where the cells are densest and therefore, arguably, more easily attacked by free radicals. While the debate seems to be swinging in favor of those experts who believe the latter area is of greater importance in causing skin to age, possibly both factors are at work. In any case, there is no doubt that free radicals do cause skin to age.

Since free radicals are molecules in search of another electron—which they tend to extract from an existing whole molecule—the way to avoid such damage is to "feed" these free radicals the extra electron they need. That is what antioxidants do. As we shall see later, the use of antioxidants, both topically and internally, is one of the basic requirements to maintain healthy, acne-free skin.

Some final thoughts on the subject of free radicals. Why, we may ask, have our bodies evolved to allow them to exist? In most other respects, our evolution has caused us to be highly resistant to the environment. One possible answer is that, from the standpoint of evolution, free radicals weren't a problem. Cigarette smoke and other man-generated pollutants didn't exist, so our bodies didn't evolve to fight them off. Of course, ultraviolet light existed, just as it does

CHEMICAL JARGON

Since we shall be describing chemicals with dauntingly long names, it's worthwhile to mention for the nonchemists reading this book that the reason many chemical names look so imposing when written, is that chemists have the habit of combining several words into one. In fact, these chemicals are really called, respectively, acetyl choline and di-methyl amino ethanol—simple enough descriptions of variations of choline and ethanol. (If English were written by chemists, this book would probably be called an acnecurativedescriptor!)

today. But our ancestors didn't survive long enough for ultraviolet light to do them much harm. Few people suffer from severe wrinkling before 40, and few people in our evolutionary past lived longer than that. Perhaps equally important, we doubt that our prehistoric ancestors spent much time sunning themselves to induce a tan, a lamentably widespread habit in modern civilization.

The other answer to the question of why our bodies didn't evolve to fight off free radicals is that fresh or uncooked foods contain a larger amount of antioxidants that fight free radicals than do processed foods. In many respects, modern food processing is essential for maintaining our health. For example, processing milk has largely wiped out tuberculosis, which, for most of the history of mankind, was a major killer. However, food processing does tend to reduce the amount of antioxidants we consume. Since our evolutionary ancestors lived exclusively on nonprocessed, or "whole," foods, their bodies were probably better equipped than ours to withstand free radicals. (More later about adding antioxidants to your diet, of course without the harm that would come from eating truly unprocessed—read "primitive"—foods.)

Sun Damage Starts Young

Thorstein Veblen, an early-20th-century economist, wrote *The Theory of the Leisure Class*, a book in which he proposed the principle that, when a society becomes affluent, its members feel the need to demonstrate that affluence to their peers. He called this "conspicuous consumption."

In China, wealthy men used to bind their wives' feet so that they could hardly walk, let alone work; the men thus showed the world that they were rich enough to have nonworking wives. In Victorian times, rich women in Europe and America wore corsets so tight that they could not bend at the waist and therefore could not possibly do any housework.

Of course, such trends are unconscious. Similarly (and of course also unconsciously), part of the reason we are a nation of sun worshippers is that young people in particular covet the tanned, bronze look and strive to achieve it the moment the summer sun starts to glare. Veblen would maintain that they are unconsciously demonstrating that they have enough leisure time—that is, they are rich enough—to get tanned instead of work.

Whatever the reason, the fact remains that, rich or poor, every time you lie on the beach—even if you do not get a sunburn—you are damaging your skin. Many years will pass before you see the damage, but see it you will.

In a recent survey of 10,079 youngsters, only one-third used a sunscreen.[1] Most reported having suffered at least one sunburn during the previous summer, and half had experienced multiple sunburns. Yet even those kids who had suffered felt that being burned was worthwhile if you eventually got a good tan out of it.

Continued excessive exposure to the sun not only inevitably causes wrinkling but also increases, by as much as 78 percent, the risk of developing various skin cancers in adulthood. More than one million Americans are diagnosed annually with skin cancer, and no one doubts that sun exposure is the leading cause.

While the risk of severe sunburn is much lower with the use of tanning beds, these too cause substantial amounts of skin damage and increase the cancer risk.

OTHER FUNCTIONS OF THE DERMIS

The dermis houses most of the specialized centers that give the skin its versatile usefulness. The most important of these are:

Blood vessels and lymph channels. These provide the nutrition for the whole skin system, including bringing in an extra rush of white corpuscles to heal wounds and antibodies to fight infections. (As we shall see later, this generally useful function has a downside: It actually helps to accelerate the spread of acne.)

An amazing variety of nerve endings. These include nerves that detect even the gentlest touch, others that sense heat and cold, still others that sense pain or itching, and, perhaps most remarkable of all, the Pacinian corpuscles, located deep in weight-bearing areas, which detect pressure.

Recent research has refined our understanding of how the nerves of the skin differentiate among sensations. It appears that there are two different "sets" of nerve endings in the skin: "thin" nerves, which work relatively slowly but transmit such subtle sensations as a mother's caress or a lover's stroke, and "thick" nerves, which work fast and efficiently to transmit other, rougher feelings.

"The fast fibers indicate when we are touched and how strong the touch is. The slow fibers signal the fine aspects of touch,"[2] said Hakan Olousson, a neurophysiologist at the Sahlgrenska University Hospital in Gothenburg, Sweden.

Without the thick nerves, which are more concentrated in our palms and soles than elsewhere, we would have difficulty in feeling objects we picked up or in sensing the temperature of something we touched. Without the thin fibers, which tend to be more available in sensitive areas, such as our forearms, we would not recognize a loving touch.

Sweat glands, which provide our all-important cooling system. Without these, we would rapidly overheat, with serious health consequences. Indeed, there is a rare condition in which people are born with an insufficient number of sweat glands. They suffer greatly, with their body temperatures often soaring well above the danger point.

Apocrine glands, which secrete a fluid mixture of proteins and minerals that, when exposed to air, cause our distinctive odors. In animals, the apocrine glands secrete pheromones, which are powerful sexual attractants. Whether human pheromones have any impact on our sexual attractiveness remains unproven. However, there is considerable evidence that babies recognize their mothers at least partly by smell.

Hair follicles, which generate as a hair "bulb" at the bottom of the dermis. These follicles are actually thin strands of a material very similar to that in the stratum corneum. However, they are far more complicated. On the side of each hair follicle, near its root, is a sebaceous gland, which produces sebum, lubricating the hair and leaving on it a thin, acidic coating that both protects it against most noxious bacteria and wards off many airborne pollutants. As we will discuss in detail later, it is the clogging of the passages from which these protective oils ooze out onto the skin—and the consequent buildup of and ultimate infection in the oils underneath—that is the proximate cause of acne. Of course, that doesn't explain why the passages get clogged. Innate in the answer to that question lies the essence of Dr. Dubrow's Acne Cure program.

THE SUBCUTANEOUS LAYER

Under the dermis lies a layer of fat cells, or lipocytes, called the subcutaneous layer. Its function is twofold.

Its most visible task is to serve as a reservoir for our bodies' nutritional needs. It is what stops us from starving—or losing so much energy that we would be unable to hunt for food—even if we are trapped with nothing to eat for several days. Unfortunately, in our comfortable modern world, this reservoir has a tendency to become overfilled, leading us to become fat. Unlike our deprived ancestors, we neither suffer from a lack of food nor face the need for vigorous exercise (having no saber-toothed tigers to evade). The result is that, according to the Surgeon General's 2001 report, 40 million Americans are obese, defined as being more than 30 percent over their ideal weight, and a horrifying 300,000 people die annually from their obesity.

The subcutaneous layer's second function is to insulate us from both excess cold and excess heat. Without such insulation, we would utilize far too much energy to keep warm in cold weather, and our sweat could not form and evaporate fast enough to keep us cool in really hot weather.

THE BASAL MEMBRANE

One fascinating aspect of our skin's structure that is too often ignored is the membrane that holds the epidermis firmly in place on top of the dermis. Without this double-sided, interlocking mechanism, the two layers would soon part company.

The important fact about the basal membrane with respect to acne is that scarring generally occurs only if this membrane is ruptured. If the acne has penetrated no further than the epidermis, no permanent damage is likely. However, this rule has one exception: In some dark skins, surface skin damage may cause extra pigmentation, which shows up as dark spots even before actual scarring, that is before the basal membrane is pierced.

For everyone, once the acne lesions pierce the basal membrane, some permanent scarring will occur. Fortunately, if the damage is minor, it may be hardly noticeable to the naked eye. However, if the acne has remained serious and untreated for a long time, the result may be serious scarring and pitting.

As we shall discuss in a later chapter, to some extent the scars can be removed or minimized. Still, if your acne is treated promptly, it should never progress far enough to rupture the basal membrane. Thus, it should never cause scarring.

WHY SKIN IS WHAT IT IS

Before we leave the subject of the skin in which we live, we should ponder a moment about why it has evolved into the organ we know.

Nearly all mammals, as well as humankind's immediate predecessors down the evolutionary ladder, have a full covering of body hair. They needed it as protection against the elements and against being wounded by both attacking predators and the thorns and stings of the undergrowth through which they scampered to avoid them. We can only speculate that, during man's evolution, as he learned to live in shelters, wear disposable skins for warmth, and avoid attack, that hair became a disadvantage. Perhaps it inhibited movement; perhaps it harbored lice. Or perhaps, once it was no longer needed for warmth (but in the absence of today's air-conditioning, swimming pools, and cold showers), it inhibited sweat from evaporating fast enough to provide maximum cooling. After all, most fur-bearing mammals crawl into the shade and limit their activity during the hottest part of the day. Or, as Noel Coward put it, "Mad dogs and Englishmen go out in the midday sun"!

For whatever reason, it is clear that eventually bare-skinned humans evolved. Even today, however, hair remains where it is needed: under arms, where it acts as a cushion to avoid chafing; in the pubic area, where it serves as a protective pad; and on the head, where it provides added protection against ultraviolet light, and cushions possible blows. In many older men, the hair no longer provides head protection. Evolutionarily, with a life expectancy of probably no more than 30 or 40, adult males would typically have been dead before this became a problem.

As we evolved, we were far less sanitary creatures than today's hygiene demands. Even in historical times, washing was hardly popular. Victorians thought that getting wet was bad for their health. And earlier, Queen Elizabeth I hardly ever took a bath. She, like her contemporaries, wore a horsehair bag near her pubic area to attract fleas that apparently prefer horse to human hair. Thus, the self-cleaning and largely self-sterilizing qualities of our skin were vital to our survival.

There may even be some cruel irony in acne. Perhaps, in the absence of marriage laws and birth control pills, even acne was of some evolutionary importance. Just conceivably, by ensuring that callow youths capable of siring and bearing children but not yet mature enough to feed or raise them were less attracted to one another, acne played some role in our human heritage.

Today, of course, acne is nothing but a physical and psychological bane. Fortunately, if we follow the precepts laid out in the following chapters, it is one that can be almost entirely avoided.

2

THE CURSE OF ACNE

VIRTUALLY 100 PERCENT OF BOYS and 90 percent of girls suffer from acne at least occasionally.[1] But men and women of all ages can be affected so that, even if you were among the lucky few who missed the curse of acne as teenagers, you may still run into trouble later. Indeed, more than 50 percent of people over 25 experience acne breakouts well into their forties and beyond.

Acne can break out anywhere on your body that pilosebaceous follicles are present—that is, just about anywhere except the palms of your hands and the soles of your feet. Obviously, however, the most common locations are face, neck, chest, and back, with the most frequent of all being the forehead, nose, lower cheeks, and chin. These, of course, are also the most visible areas and therefore the most disturbing to sufferers.

Moreover, the problem is not merely physical: Young people and old, men and women, often experience psychological trauma and real heartache from their acne. Even when it isn't so bad, people often *feel* terrible about themselves. In his clinical practice, Dr. Dubrow hears their heartfelt complaints.

"I can't ask girls out," an 18-year-old boy confided to him. Admittedly, the young man had some pimples on his chin, but his condition was not terrible, and otherwise he was healthy and attractive. No doubt many a girl would have been delighted with him. But he was convinced, "They'll think I'm a zit freak." And nothing would change his mind until, using the Acne Cure, his acne disappeared.

"I'm scared to accept invitations to go out," said a woman who had become a virtual recluse. "I'm shy by nature. And as soon as I accept an invitation, I get nervous and anxious, and then the most horrible outbreak of acne appears. It happens just about every time." Although the acne was not nearly as severe as she assumed, she was correct in observing that as soon as she became stressed by the combination of an impending anxiety-producing social event and the expectation of an acne attack, her acne did flare up. Since she was convinced that there was nothing she could do about it, the stress became that much worse; the vicious circle drew tighter.

"I look horrible," an attractive 30-year-old woman complained. In fact, her "horrible" skin consisted of no more than some whiteheads on her nose and a larger, infected pimple on her forehead. But to her, that pimple was a beacon, as distracting as an additional eye staring out just above her nose.

"I don't think I'll make partner," stated a 36-year-old lawyer whose face was covered with relatively mild acne. "The acne. It makes me look like an overgrown kid. They'll think I lack maturity." Nothing could convince this very accomplished professional that acne was not a career-ender.

As with many of Dr. Dubrow's patients, these four self-assessments were far harsher than the facts warranted. Nevertheless, that's how they felt. After all, they reasoned, if they found their acne to be dreadful, why wouldn't others feel the same? This view holds some logic, however flawed, and is therefore hard to dispel.

Feelings of this sort do grievous harm to anyone's life, self-image, and happiness. On several occasions, we have heard about acne sufferers who became so depressed about their acne—and the negative effects it had on their lives—that they had seriously contemplated suicide.

When dermatologists and other physicians confront acne severe enough to give rise to suicidal feelings, they often move straight to prescribing the most drastic anti-acne medicine of all, Accutane (about which we will write in more detail later). It works to eliminate almost all acne (including most of the 5 percent Dr. Dubrow's program doesn't fully resolve). However, it can have serious side effects, including bleeding gums, dry mouth and cracked lips, enhanced sun sensitivity, hair loss, headaches, and dried nasal linings, which may lead to nosebleeds. It may also cause birth defects and should therefore never be used by women who are or shortly intend to become pregnant.

Obviously, a patient who is brought to thoughts of suicide by acne is likely to suffer more generally from depression as well. No doubt the acne aggravates those feelings, but it is likely not their only cause. Thus, the alleviation of depression that may result from eliminating acne by taking Accutane may be offset, at least in part, by other physical problems caused by the Accutane. These, in turn, may affect the underlying depression.

While many people feel more unhappy about their acne than the symptoms seem to justify, it is also true that for many sufferers acne is so disfiguring that they may be on the mark in believing that their appearance is aversive to others. If severe acne is left untreated, it can leave permanent scars to mar an otherwise handsome or beautiful face.

There are three basic types of acne scars:

1. The most common type—and the least severe—is generally referred to as *ice picks*. It is due to the loss of part of the epidermis so that the skin "dimples" slightly.

2. The second type of scar, called *craters*, occurs when the epidermis is "captured" by the scar tissue of a deeper acne lesion and is pulled into a deeper pit.

3. In some cases, especially on darker or Black skin, acne spots may turn into *keloids*, which are almost like flat warts raised on the surface of the skin. Initially red and itchy, they eventually become hard and dark. They can grow to several centimeters in diameter.

No scars are easy to remove, but, as we shall discuss later, there is quite a lot that can be done to minimize their visibility. The best course by far is to cure your acne before scarring ever becomes a problem.

Millions of acne sufferers endure the physical and psychological effects of acne, and millions of dollars are spent trying to treat it. Until now, there has been no cure. Obviously, there is an ocean of ignorance about the disease in both the public and the medical communities.

WHY ACNE REMEDIES DON'T WORK

The reason for the ignorance and misunderstanding about acne is ironic. It is inadvertently fostered by the very commercial concerns that are spending hundreds of millions of dollars to sell acne cures.

Because acne hits virtually everyone, countless billions of dollars have been spent over the years developing, marketing, and promoting a plethora of products to deal with the problem. Why, then, do so many people continue to feel that acne is an incurable condition?

Simple: Although those products help in the treatment of acne up to a point, they don't solve the problem for most people most of the time.

As we shall discuss in the next chapter, acne is a disease that has four specific stages. For each stage, there are products available that work pretty well. However, if you use only one such product, it will cure your acne only if, by coincidence, all your acne is in the stage that particular product aims to attack. In almost all cases, though, some parts of your overall acne are in stage 1 of the disease, some in stage 2, and so on. Naturally, then, however effective a product is in attacking one of those stages, it won't work to cure the rest of your acne. You would not be correct in concluding that the product doesn't work; but you would be wholly accurate in observing that it is not, in fact, a cure.

There is another problem with the anti-acne products now on the market. This issue again carries with it a fair load of irony. For it is the very power of the skin—and especially of the stratum corneum—to ward off chemicals that makes it so difficult for acne creams and lotions to penetrate to where they are needed. Worse, when the skin is damaged—be it by a cut or abrasion or by the destructive effects of acne—your body promptly fights to repair itself. One of the ways it does that is to close up the damaged area by inflaming—and therefore swelling—the surrounding skin. The closure makes it that much more difficult for the healing ointments to penetrate and do any good.

This lack of penetration renders most products less effective than they should be, leaving many with little or no effectiveness at all—and leaving you feeling that you've wasted your money.

THE REAL HARM OF ACNE:
SCARRING THE SOUL

It is the psychological impact of acne—and of the scarring that occurs if it is severe and left untreated—that is the real harm done by the disease. Kelly Bartlett, apparently a young teenager, posted a poem about acne on the Internet. Called "Pubescent Lament," it includes the lines:

Oh, why must I experience this horrible pubescent pain?

I can't remember the last time I felt such shame.[2]

The conviction that acne is incurable is so widespread that there is even a worldwide support group (the Acne Support Group), headquartered in England, to help sufferers live with their disfiguring acne.[3] Its 6,000 members talk to one another about how bad their problem makes them feel, about how their pimples make them feel suicidal, about how their parents don't or didn't understand their disease, about how their love lives were destroyed by their skin condition—in net, about how awful their lives are as a result of their acne. In the introduction of a work commissioned by the Acne Support Group, Anthony C. Chu, M.D., F.R.C.P., consultant dermatologist to the Imperial College of Science, Technology and Medicine at the Hammersmith Hospital in England, stated, "Acne is . . . a stigma that sufferers must bear—something to be ashamed of, something to be ridiculed about."[4]

Later, Dr. Chu stated, "All treatments [of acne] should give at least 50 percent response in the first two months of therapy."[5] That presumably leaves the other 50 percent with acne that doesn't respond to treatment, or at least not within a reasonable time. No wonder Dr. Chu describes some of his patients as taking down all the mirrors in their homes so that they won't see themselves. No wonder too that he has a patient who "would lie in bed and feel her face to see how many spots had come up overnight before even getting out of bed."[6]

The acne Web site of the American Academy of Dermatology, AcneNet, asks, "What should you do with the psychological and emotional effects of acne?" Their answer is in five steps. The first three of them—which we have shortened here—are:

1. *Don't try to deny that acne might have a negative effect on your life.*

2. Learn the facts about the causes and cures of acne. If you learn the facts, it will be clear that acne is never your fault.

3. Help your parents and friends learn the facts about acne. A supportive family is one of your most important resources for building and maintaining self-esteem.[7]

WHY SUFFER FROM A CURABLE DISEASE?

All this suffering about acne makes us furious. The truth is:

Your acne problems can be solved;
you don't have to suffer!

Why should your life be devastated by a skin condition that, in 95 percent of cases, can be cured at little cost within 6 weeks—and usually in a lot less time? Why should you be concerned about the negative reaction people will have to your "horrible" skin condition when you can have lovely skin? Why should you be stigmatized or ridiculed? If any ridicule is in order, it should be reserved for people who perpetuate the myth that acne is an inevitable condition, something you have to live with. You *don't*!

Usually, once you have beaten your acne, it won't come back. Oh, sure, once in a while you may get an occasional pimple. This is especially so if you're experiencing sudden high stress or there is an abrupt change in your hormonal structure—for example, if you become pregnant. But a single pimple—even if it seems the size of Mount Vesuvius—that lasts only a few days and (provided you quickly reinstate the Acne Cure program) is not going to be the precursor of a full-blown acne attack is hardly going to destroy your life or give you suicidal feelings. Having a nasty, unsightly rash all over your face may well reduce your chances of getting a date or getting promoted. But a single, occasional pimple won't put anybody off, at least not anyone worth having.

Of course, the Academy of Dermatology knows that acne, properly treated, need not be a problem. They know—as stated on their AcneNet site—that "most" types of acne can be "effectively treated."[8] But the rest of the site seems unconnected to this accurate statement. For, if acne can in fact be eradicated in almost every case, why does this Web site comment on the emotional and social trauma of acne? No one suffers trauma from an easily treatable disease!

The Web site stated correctly, "Just about every case of acne can be cleared up, but sometimes it takes a dermatologist's help." Technically, that is true. However, the implication is that eliminating the disease generally requires a specialist's intervention, which can be expensive and time-consuming. On the contrary, the truth is that the vast majority of acne cases—including many severe ones—can be eradicated by following the program we shall describe shortly.

AcneNet then provided the basic treatment protocol. Just listen to two of the "requirements":

- **"Don't pop your acne."** Okay. We emphatically agree with this. But who can avoid popping out some huge whitehead? Our view is that you shouldn't pop—that is, unless you use the services of a physician or certified aesthetician with appropriate instruments. But in the real world, the only effective way to stop yourself from doing so is to *avoid* the "poppable" pimple in the first place.

- **"Avoid things like . . . airborne grease . . . and [rough or tight] sporting equipment."** Come on! What happens if you live in the real world, where airborne everything is unavoidable? Of course, it would be better for our health—including the health of our skin and the likelihood of suffering from acne—if we lived in cleaner air than many of us now experience. But we don't. And the gradual improvements in our environment resulting from the Clean Air Act and public pressure take place too slowly to have an effect on our current condition. Anyhow, what happens to teenagers who flip burgers in a fast-food joint to augment their pocket money? Or to the short-order cook in our favorite diner who spends his entire shift splattered with grease? Are they doomed to terminal acne? And what if you want to exercise healthfully? We never yet met a piece of gym equipment that was loose and velvet soft! And does that also mean that we have to give up our favorite spandex outfit in favor of baggy clothing?

The rest of the advice was fine, but the fact is, you don't need to follow it to get rid of your acne. It's not wrong; it's just largely unnecessary.

By the way, if you have to spend your life in a McDonald's kitchen, rest assured that, whatever else it may do to your health, as long as you follow the steps we recommend, the acne you may have now will disappear, and you will be able to live essentially acne-free forever.

TYPES OF ACNE

There are several different types of acne. By far the most common—the one that accounts for some 95 percent of all acne—is called *acne vulgaris*. That is the one that the procedure outlined in this book will eradicate.

Other types of acne may be tougher to deal with—but even they can be largely eliminated by the method we will outline. This is because the more esoteric acnes are usually found in conjunction with acne vulgaris. Therefore, the two (or more) forms of the disease tend to aggravate each other medically, visually, and psychologically. Thus, by eliminating the vulgaris portion of the problem, you will have already made considerable progress in eliminating the whole problem.

The remainder of the problem—that portion of it caused by the less tractable forms of acne—requires medications that may cause other difficulties. Thus, you may need a dermatologist to look at some of these other types of the disease. We will deal with all these issues—applicable to only a tiny percentage of the readers of this book—in chapter 11. So here's a suggestion . . .

Try implementing the Acne Cure program as soon as you have completed reading chapter 4. Then read the rest of the book, but skip chapter 11. In other words, don't worry yet about dealing with those acnes the protocol outlined in chapter 4 won't completely eliminate.

Assuming it takes you a while to finish the book, you may well find that by the time you get around to reading chapter 11, your "incurable" acne will have disappeared, that it was not as intractable as you thought! Or, if you are a fast reader, you may see that your acne, while not yet fully eradicated, has been greatly reduced. In that case, keep going with our cure protocol for the whole 6 weeks to see if your acne disappears. The beauty of this approach is that, even if the Acne Cure program doesn't entirely clear up your acne and you therefore still feel you need a dermatologist, he or she will be able to get straight to the heart of the problem without having to deal with vulgaris before moving on to the tough stuff.

OVERSIMPLIFYING ACNE

In its simplest terms, the development of acne is easy to describe. A channel from which a hair follicle has emerged or is about to emerge becomes blocked. The sebaceous gland attached to the lower part of that follicle continues to produce its oily sebum. But since the clog stops the sebum from emerging, it stays inside the channel and expands into a balloon full of the stuff. Before long, the sebum—warm, oily, and nutritious—attracts bacteria and starts to putrefy. The result is a nasty pimple. Eventually, the pressure builds up so much that the pimple bursts and the mess erupts onto your skin. Or, worse, the clog may stay in place and the "balloon" may rupture inward. That is what nearly always happens, at least in part, when you try to pop a pimple. In either case, you are obviously helping to spread the germs to any other spots of sebum buildup—and, so, encouraging them to become infected more quickly.

However, that is only the short version of how acne proceeds. It is the form many experts, articles, and books describe, and it is therefore the description many people recognize. But, while not wrong, it is a dangerous oversimplification. Because this "short form" explanation sounds so seductively simple and logical, it leads to the view that a simple solution (slather on something like Clearasil) should solve the problem. As we have explained, more often than not, the simple solution doesn't work. For the fact is that the progress of acne—and particularly the mechanism of its spread—is a good deal more complicated. And because it is, it needs a more sophisticated regimen to cure it. The next chapter details what acne is and how it develops.

3

WHAT IS ACNE?
HOW IS IT GENERATED?
HOW DOES IT SPREAD?

IN COMPLICATED SCIENTIFIC PARLANCE, acne is caused by abnormal desquamation of follicular epithelium that results in the obstruction of the pilosebaceous canal. Actually the facts are simple. There are four contributory factors that lead to acne.

1. The oily mixture called sebum—produced by the sebaceous glands attached to the hair follicles near the base of your pores—normally lubricates your skin to keep it healthy, soft, pliable, and protected (much as a good antiseptic moisturizer does). Sebum combines with the dead skin cells called keratinocytes to form plugs that block further sebum from emerging from your pores.

2. The sebaceous glands keep producing sebum, but because it can't escape, the sebum balloons up, trapped inside your pores.

3. Bacteria attack the trapped sebum, degrading it.

4. The inflammation that is your body's attempt to eradicate the bacteria actually helps spread the condition.

That, in a nutshell, is how most lay books and articles about acne (as well as, sadly, some less than fully informed physicians) describe the disease. As a result, while this description is not actually incorrect, it is woefully *incomplete* and, by oversimplifying the disease, gives sufferers the wrong idea about how to deal with it.

For example, if you knew no more than the above summary about acne, you would conclude that coating your skin with a bacteria-fighting antiseptic would quickly clear up the condition. After all, if acne occurs only in the presence of bacteria present, and you kill the bacteria, why, no more acne! There are several such antiseptic creams and ointments on the market, and they often help to some extent. Occasionally, they even eliminate the problem. More often than not, however, the acne remains.

Alternatively, again relying only on the above description, you would think that regular abrasive washing with detergents to remove loose keratinocytes would largely eliminate acne. With no dead skin cells around, there should be nothing to mix with the sebum to form a plug. Right?

No! Not only would you be wrong, but you would actually be aggravating your condition.

And again, if the problem is that your pores are plugged up, then surely a good abrasive scrub would get rid of the plugs and do wonders for your acne. Again, this is dangerously incorrect. Harsh or abrasive cleansing is among the worst things you can do for your condition.

Clearly, then, we need a fuller explanation. There are four stages in acne, three that concern its formation and a fourth that concerns its spread. Let us discuss each of these in turn.

STAGE 1

As we described in chapter 1, your skin replaces itself almost completely, depending on your age, every 28 to 45 days. That is its highly effective way of avoiding the buildup of the damage done to it day in and day out by ultraviolet light, pollution, and general wear and tear. In this process, dead keratinocytes on your skin's surface—that is, the stratum corneum—are sloughed off, and new cells from the base of the epidermis work their way up to replace them.

When this process works correctly, the old cells on the surface of the stratum corneum fall off uniformly, and new flattened cells are added from below at the same rate. However, sometimes (for a variety of reasons we will discuss shortly) your body suddenly produces an excess of sebum. Since the sebum is oily and somewhat sticky, it may combine with some of the loose cells at the surface of the stratum corneum so that instead of sloughing off, they produce a paste-like material. This paste may then wedge itself into an open hair follicle (pore) and there set, compact, and harden into a solid, hard-to-remove wad that partially plugs up the mouth of the pore.

At the same time, there appears to be a change in the constitution of the cells that line the hair follicle canal, and this may be an even greater problem than the surface plugs. Apparently, through a series of hormonal events that scientists do not fully understand, some or all of these internal cells become sticky. Normally, as they dry, the cells lining the follicle are swept out by the emerging sebum. But once they become sticky as a result of those hormonal or other changes, the sebum can no long rinse them out. Instead, they adhere to the sides of the canal, adding to the partial blockage.

These partial blockages are called microcomedones. The first impact of these microcomedones is that they force the canal to dilate, which enlarges the pores at the skin's surface, a condition typical of acne sufferers. Apart from their looking unattractive, these enlarged pores are something of a mixed blessing. On the one hand, they allow more of the sebum to emerge, thus delaying or reducing the amount of internal sebum buildup. On the other hand, the larger mouths of the pores are more likely to gather plugs from the cell-and-sebum mixture on the surface of the stratum corneum.

As more sebum builds up inside the pore, if the partial blockage is generated from the external "paste" of cells and sebum and is therefore near the surface, you start to see blackheads. The dark color of blackheads comes from a pigment in the sebum, not from dirt. Nevertheless, they look "dirty" and are unsightly.

If the blockage is generated by sticky internal cells and is therefore further down the canal, you will see only a slight reddening and a bump. An acne spot is sure to erupt eventually, but so far it is still too far down to be visible. In profusion, these deep down microcomedones give rise to the bumpy feel of the skin even when the acne has not yet broken out.

Next, sweat penetrates past the partial blockage into the stagnant sebum and, through a series of chemical and physical reactions, turns it into a waxy, "cheesy" consistency. This is what you see emerging if you (unwisely) squeeze your acne spots. The water in the sweat also causes the canal walls to swell, much as the skin on your fingers swells if you keep them too long in water. Generally, this mild swelling is desirable, as it keeps the skin healthfully moisturized. However, in this special case, the moisture tends to further occlude the pores, thus wedging in the wads and blocking the pores even tighter.

Before long—between the internal "sticky" cells of the canal, the external cell-and-sebum "cement," and the water-swollen canal itself—a complete blockage occurs. This so-called comedone may appear either as a firm white pustule or whitehead (called a closed comedone) or as an expanded blackhead (called an open comedone). In either case, the plug is now so firmly in place that no sebum can escape at all. And your skin is ready for the next, really nasty stage of acne.

STAGE 2

While all this is happening, your sebaceous gland, near the bottom of the follicular canal (or pore), is still in full swing, unaffected by the existence of a plug closer to or at the canal's exit. Consequently, with nowhere to go, the sebum starts to build up and expand the canal. Eventually, it forms a small internal balloon. This is what you feel when those red spots swell and become sore to the touch. The sorer they are, the larger the sebum balloon and the more certain you are that a nasty zit is on the way.

There are several occasions when the body may produce more sebum than usual. The most important is when the sudden generation of testosterone, a condition that all males and females experience during puberty, activates the sebaceous glands. We don't fully understand how testosterone—produced by the testes in men and by the adrenal glands (situated just above the kidneys) in women—sensitizes the sebaceous glands to produce more sebum. However, we do know that it is not the amount of testosterone that determines how much acne forms. Rather, any new spurt of testosterone production stimulates the production of excess sebum.

If the amount of testosterone were determinant, men would obviously suffer far more from acne than women, and acne sufferers would have larger amounts of testosterone in their systems than non-sufferers. Moreover, one noted side effect of men who are placed on a testosterone supplement regime—a somewhat controversial therapy that some physicians prescribe to improve muscle tone, bone density, and libido—would be the appearance of acne. None of this is true. Thus, acne is certainly not a hormonal disease.

Another frequent trigger of acne in both men and women is stress (which we will discuss in detail in chapter 10). Again, we are not certain exactly how stress causes the production of more sebum, although there are several plausible theories. But no doubt there is a connection. Indeed, a not infrequent phenomenon is the appearance of acne in brides just before the wedding date—at precisely the moment they least want their faces to break out! This is stress-induced acne. And of course the acne adds to the stress and thus tends to perpetuate itself.

In women, a third important influence on acne is the hormonal changes associated with the menstrual cycle, during which testosterone and other hormones experience significant variations not only in quantity but also in the way they affect various bodily functions and feelings. Similarly, acne is often influenced by the onset of pregnancy or birth. A newly pregnant woman may paradoxically find that her acne suddenly clears up completely or suddenly reappears after years of absence. Then, when she has had her baby, she may again experience an onset or a cessation of her acne. Even more annoying, there is no guarantee that the problem always goes in opposite directions. Quite possibly, it could get worse both at the onset and at the completion of pregnancy. No one ever said having babies is easy!

Fortunately, the Acne Cure program will work just fine for pregnant women. And, because it involves no ingested drugs, and only very well proven external medications, there is no doubt in our minds that it is as safe for them as for anyone else. Nevertheless, if you are pregnant, before using these (or any) medications, even externally, you should first check with your obstetrician.

The first symptom of an overstimulated sebaceous gland is unusually oily skin. Teenage boys, in particular, seem to suffer from this condition. Among other symptoms, this gives rise to the lank, oily hair that has become almost a trademark of teenage idols. Contrary to many a parent's incorrect belief, the condition has little to do with poor personal hygiene.

Oily skin is not in itself unhealthy. On the contrary, at a time when teenage boys' hair follicle growth is in full swing—and the skin's pores therefore open and the stratum corneum still relatively thin—the extra oil may provide valuable protection. Moreover, extra oil in adults tends to fight all sorts of the aging effects, including the formation of wrinkles and the development of dry, gray skin that we associate with either poor health or advancing age. However, excess oil production (especially among teenagers) carries with it the disadvantage that, combined with the rapidly shedding skin cells, it is available to form the plugs that can easily clog open pores.

STAGE 3

Even though healthy skin is protected from excessive levels of bacteria by the sebum covering it, we all carry, both on the skin's surface and inside our pores, a safe level of many different types of bacteria. Among those is a little fellow called *Propionibacterium acnes* or, fittingly enough, *P. acnes* for short. It is a hearty character, tough to kill both because it is resistant to many bacteriocides and because it lives not only on the skin's surface but also hidden deep within your pores.

Normally, *P. acnes* is kept under control both because the sebum tends to leach out excessive growths of the bacteria from your pores and because the sebum is mildly acidic, a condition *P. acnes* dislikes. However, once the sebum builds up in a static balloon, the *P. acnes*, now living in a warm, damp, oily "broth" of sebum, is able to overcome (or perhaps neutralize) the acidity and multiply in profusion. The result is that the sebum degrades and turns into an infected, suppurating mixture of oil and pus.

Among other unpleasant effects of this mess is its tendency to breed bacteria and generate toxins that attack the canal walls, thinning and weakening them. Since they are already stretched, this obviously heightens the risk of their rupture.

Eventually, of course, the mess has to break out. It does so either by spewing onto the surface of the skin or, if you are unlucky, by breaking inward. This occurs if the canal walls have thinned enough, if the surface plug is particularly thick and firmly fixed, if the pus balloon is extra deep, or if there is a combination of all of these. When it does happen, you suffer from a deep, sore lump in your skin that may not subside for several weeks. If the condition is severe enough, a new infection may occur deep inside your epidermis and may form a cyst that will pierce the barrier membrane and penetrate deep into the dermis. When that happens, you are likely to have a permanent scar.

By the way, this also explains why it is so undesirable to squeeze your pimples. Because you cannot squeeze them entirely from underneath, if you do squeeze, you are likely to push some of the pus down into the dermis as well as up and out. If that happens (and it is almost bound to if you squeeze frequently), you are not only prolonging your condition but also, even worse, risking the formation of acne cysts, which cause permanent scarring. Under certain conditions your medical practitioner may "squeeze" a particularly nasty acne lesion as an alternative to removing it surgically. However, he or she will use a special instrument designed to remove the material without rupturing the canal. There is no way you can duplicate this procedure at home.

STAGE 4

The final stage (perhaps the most interesting, and certainly the most misunderstood) explains how acne spreads.

The first step in the spread of acne represents another irony, namely that the spread of acne is partly caused by the body's own defense mechanism against the invasion of *P. acnes*. What happens is that, in fighting off this bacterial attack, your body sends to the scene extra blood carrying white corpuscles and various antibodies. This accounts for much of the redness of inflammation. To some extent this reaction is effective as that particular pimple eventually goes away.

However, the extra "curative" blood has an unfortunate side effect: It swells the surrounding areas, squeezing the pores, making them more susceptible to clogging and tending to turn partially blocked pores into full-fledged comedones that harbor the bacteria that have been breeding nearby. Thus, while curing one acne pimple, the inflammation actually facilitates the formation of many more.

As you can see, the process of the formation of acne is clear: Dry cells mixed with sebum block the pores; sebum builds up behind the clog; bacteria infect the buildup; and the eventual "curative" inflammation spreads the condition.

The goals of the Acne Cure program, then, become obvious. It has to:

1. Avoid the clogging

2. Remove both the clogs and the excess collected sebum from already clogged pores

3. Kill the bacteria inside and outside those pores

4. Stop the inflammation so as to avoid spreading the condition.

In principle, taking these four steps should be simple enough. And in practice it is . . . once you know how. But learning how to implement such a program is not at all simple. Dr. Dubrow has worked on the problem for years and only recently perfected a program that fully attacks all four parts.

Once Dr. Dubrow had perfected the program, he still faced the task of persuading sufferers to follow it—and so eradicate the disease. This task was complicated by two factors. The first is that the causes of and cure for acne are surrounded by any number of myths and old wives' tales, often fervently believed but mostly wrong.

The other, as we have emphasized earlier, is that the dozens of commercial acne products—marketed with huge sums to tout their efficacy—foster a state of misinformation, or at least incomplete information, about acne. Many of the advertised products work up to a point and therefore have their convinced advocates. But none works for all sufferers all the time because each attacks only one or at most two of the four causes of acne. Thus, they are effective only when a user's acne happens to be caused primarily by the condition the specific medication attacks.

As Dr. Dubrow has observed in his practice time and again, acne sufferers respond to this lack of apparent effectiveness in a number of ways, each of which is largely counterproductive.

The first and most usual way is that, believing the old wives' tale that acne is caused by dirt, they start washing their skin with ever more vigor. Often they use soaps or various exfoliants that strip the surface of the skin with mildly abrasive granules, such as crushed peach pits or powdered pumice. We doubt that these abrasives do anyone much good; however, we are sure that they can damage acned skin. You should avoid them at all costs.

As long as we're on the subject, let us emphasize that abrasion is never desirable for skin except when conducted by an aesthetician, a dermatologist, or a plastic surgeon skilled in the technique. If you self-abrade, you may do some damage to your healthy skin, though you will not succeed in removing unwanted dry skin or doing anything else worthwhile. In fact, as we have explained, the main result of overvigorous skin cleaning is more dried-out and flaky skin, and a consequent worsening of your acne.

The next step unrelieved acne sufferers take is to either slather on whatever product they are using or switch to products with higher concentrations of the active ingredient. Such reactions, while understandable, are contraindicated. At best, they constitute a waste of money. If a product isn't working because it is not designed to attack the particular stage of acne from which you are suffering, using more of it won't make it work any better. At worst, using more may even do some harm. For example, benzoyl peroxide, one of the ingredients in the Acne Cure program, reaches its maximum effectiveness between 2.5% and 5.0%. However, there are products on the market with concentrations as high as 10%. These cost more and, on sensitive skin (or skin sensitized by acne lesions), may cause a nasty burning sensation.

When nothing else works, sufferers' final response to what they regard as their intractable condition is to see a physician (who may or may not be a specialist in the disease). By this time, of course, patients are likely to be distraught by their "horrible" acne (which their attempts to cure may have aggravated). In too many cases, influenced by their patients' concern, physicians overreact by prescribing antibiotics or Accutane (an ineffective and sometimes dangerous drug that we shall discuss below).

In rare cases, truly intractable acne may justify the use of these powerful drugs in spite of their cost and potentially serious side effects. However, as we shall describe in chapter 11, they should be used only in the very rare instance when our Acne Cure program has been fully implemented yet the acne still persists.

Side effects from antibiotics fall into three categories:

1. Some patients complain of immediate unpleasant side effects such as severe headaches from tetracycline, dizziness from minocyline, and increased sun sensitivity from both.

2. Antibiotics destroy some microorganisms more efficiently than others, changing the bacterial balance in our bodies. As a result, some of these microorganisms, usually kept in check by "enemy" bacteria, may find that enemy weakened and therefore have the chance to grow unchecked. For example, many women who use tetracycline find that they fall victim to vaginal yeast infections.

3. Finally, there is a longer-term problem which may prove to be more serious than the other two. The bacteria in our bodies tend to "learn" how to withstand specific antibiotics by evolving new strains that are resistant to them. Thus, if you use such drugs unnecessarily(for instance, to eliminate acne that can be easily cured by simpler means), you may remove a potential cure for a much more serious disease. Indeed, indiscriminate use of antibiotics has been widely decried by many leading physicians. Nevertheless, antibiotics remain widely prescribed for acne. For example, an estimated 10 percent of all tetracycline sold in the United States is prescribed for that purpose.

Even more draconian than antibiotics is the "ultimate" acne cure, namely Accutane (isotretinoin). This is a highly effective but somewhat dangerous drug of last resort. It works by inhibiting the production of sebum, and it is almost magically effective against even the most severe acne. However, it has two side effects, one of which is exceedingly important because, if ignored, it can cause devastating problems.

One side effect applies to pregnant women: *Accutane taken during pregnancy can cause birth defects.*

Obviously, Accutane should not be used by any woman who is pregnant or who intends to become so. A woman taking Accutane should not allow herself to become pregnant until at least 2 months after ending the use of this drug.

Admittedly, the risk of a birth defect due to Accutane, while real, is not large. And if a woman carefully practices birth control while taking Accutane, the risk of an unplanned pregnancy is small. Thus, the danger that a baby might be born with a birth defect resulting from the use of Accutane is also very small. Nevertheless, we recommend against the use of Accutane by sexually active women of childbearing age who would be unwilling to terminate a pregnancy.

The less problematic but sometimes still unpleasant side effects of Accutane have to do with a reduction in sebum production—the very method by which Accutane is effective against acne. Reduced sebum may result in severely dry skin, leading to nosebleeds, cracked lips, bleeding gums, a raspy throat, and other discomforts. Accutane can also cause more general symptoms such as headaches and occasionally even musculoskeletal problems. All of these are generally (but not always) mild. And they all cease as soon as the Accutane is discontinued.

In summary, then, rather than fret about your acne—and certainly before you resort to the use of antibiotics, Accutane, or other prescription drugs—we urge you to try the Acne Cure program described in detail in the next chapter.

In order to cure acne, all four phases of the disease must be eliminated. Once this is understood, and the cause of acne and the method by which it spreads is clear, the Acne Cure program Dr. Dubrow has developed will seem so logical as to appear almost self-evident. We hope that, as a result, millions of men and women of all ages who now suffer from acne will learn how to apply the program and overcome their acne problems. We hope and believe that, rather than learning to live with their acne, this book will teach them how to live happily without it.

4

THE ACNE CURE PROGRAM

ONCE YOU FULLY UNDERSTAND THE CAUSES
and development of acne, you will find the Acne Cure program logical, obvious, relatively simple—and remarkably reliable.

After following the program outlined in this chapter for 6
weeks (and often for much less time), 95 out of 100
people will find that their acne has vanished.

The art of the Acne Cure program lies in the fact that each of the
four stages of your acne, although treated concurrently, is handled
with its own medication, as if it were a separate disease. So if you
follow this program, your acne doesn't stand much of a chance.

Once your acne has disappeared, it will generally stay away as
long as you follow a simple, four-step maintenance program. This will
be described in detail in chapter 6, Beautiful Skin. The chapter title is
apropos because the program does more than just maintain your skin
in good condition; it actually helps to rejuvenate your skin, often with
the effect of making it (and therefore you) look years younger.

In some cases, your acne may start to reappear (although usually
in far milder form than originally). Don't worry; just revert to the full
Acne Cure program for a few days, and the acne will disappear again.
Alternatively, if you know you are about to face a particularly tense
time (for example, if you are in the final countdown to your wedding

day, or if you have decided to seek a new job and you have an important interview coming up), you may want to use the program prophylactically to stop the acne from ever showing up. Either way, once you have cured your acne for the first time, you will have little difficulty either in keeping it away or, if it does show up, in quickly beating it into renewed submission.

A large majority of even the 5 percent of sufferers who are affected by the far rarer, and in some cases tougher, forms of acne will see their condition improved. As we have mentioned before, this is because the more difficult forms of acne are nearly always combined with the standard version of the disease, the one that can be completely eradicated. (We will address in chapter 11 how to eliminate whatever acne may remain after you have completed the program.)

Before we go into detail about each of the steps of the Acne Cure program, let us summarize the principle of how it works.

1. To minimize the spread of acne, you obviously need to cleanse the skin as much as practical, *without* drying it out excessively. Dry skin will shed a greater portion of its stratum corneum and thus have more flaky material available to mix with the same amount of sebum emerging from the follicular canals. It will therefore be more, not less, likely to cause clogging plugs.

Incidentally, regular toilet soap is less than ideal as a skin-cleansing agent because it is by nature somewhat alkaline and therefore tends to neutralize sebum's acidic—and hence antibacterial—properties. Neutral-pH cleansing creams and nonsoap "beauty bars" are better.

2. Next you need to remove the plugs that are already clogging the pores. Removing those relatively close to the surface is not difficult. The harder trick is to get the ones forming deep down.

To some extent, of course, there is nothing to be done about really deep and fully closed comedones. If all you see is a red lump with no entrance, nothing short of surgery will reach down deep enough to attack the balloon of sebum and pus that is slowly forming and expanding way down there. You simply have to let the body do its work, allow the pimple to appear and eventually erupt. Of course, in the meantime, you have to stop any new comedones from forming. That is why in severe cases the Acne Cure program may take up to 6 weeks to become fully effective—that is, for the last deep infection to reach the surface and clear up. However, during that time, as the deep bumps sequentially reach the surface and no new ones form, you will see your acne getting better and less visible day by day.

3. This step is in some ways the most difficult. Remember, it is the inflammation itself—that is, the body's attempt to cure itself—that swells up the area around the pores and thus causes them to close all the more tightly. Therefore, the trick in this stage is to eliminate the inflammation so that the pores open up enough to get a curative medication down inside them, where it is needed to clear up the infection.

However, while we want to reduce the inflammation and the swelling that goes with it, we don't want to interrupt the body's own ability to cure infections. Those white corpuscles rushing to the scene are valuable in the curative process.

Achieving this rather contradictory result—that is, bringing in extra blood without causing the undesirable swelling—might sound complicated. The process is simpler than you would imagine. Simple, but nevertheless vital to achieving full success.

4. The final step in the Acne Cure program is not directly about curing acne. It is about making sure the skin remains healthy, largely wrinkle-free, and not prone to the recurrence of the disease. While there is no proof, we are convinced that healthy, vibrant skin is less likely to fall prey to acne than is poorly maintained skin. Healthy skin's stratum corneum will be smoother, its pores smaller, its sebum

production more regular, and the incidence of "sticky" cell production less frequent. All this suggests that acne is less likely to strike. Research to support this contention would be difficult to do—and none has been attempted. But the proposition seems reasonable, and it is consistent with the experience of Dr. Dubrow's patients.

In any case, maintaining *healthy* skin is the same as maintaining young-looking, wrinkle-free skin—and who doesn't want that?

There, those are the principles of the Acne Cure program. It's logical; and it works. So now let's delve into each of the four steps in more detail.

STEP 1

CLEANING AWAY EXCESS DEAD CELLS

The old adage that an ounce of prevention is worth a pound of cure applies here. Therefore, the first step in the Acne Cure program is to clean off the excess dead cells from the skin's surface while also killing any bacteria that may be entrenched there, ready to attack.

Of course, this step must not dry out the skin. Sebum provides a valuable protective layer to the skin that works effectively to protect it against many of the pathogenic bacteria and fungi that would otherwise attack it.

Moreover, as we emphasized previously, removing the sebum from the surface of the skin does not stop the sebaceous glands from producing it. Remember, clogs form when dry skin cells—either in the pores themselves or on the skin's surface, next to the pores—combine with the emerging sebum. By drying the skin's surface, excessive washing makes more dry skin cells available to combine with the emerging sebum. Thus, it has the opposite effect from the one you are trying to achieve.

The best ingredient by far for this preliminary cleaning and sanitizing is salicylic acid, a product that is widely available in commercial brands sold in your drugstore or supermarket. As a matter of fact, salicylic acid (the base for aspirin, by the way) is an interesting chemical. In addition to being an excellent first step in your acne treatment, it has two other important benefits.

One is that it is an anti-inflammatory. Thus, while it is washing the surface of your skin, it has a tendency also to reduce the swelling around the pores and, so, is able to penetrate at least a little into those microcomedones that are starting to cause pimples.

The second benefit of salicylic acid is that it is a special form of antioxidant. Using antioxidants is a mainstay of keeping skin youthful and wrinkle-free. While many dermatologists believe that salicylic acid is not technically an antioxidant, Nicholas Perricone, M.D., in his book *The Wrinkle Cure* stated, "Not only does it scoop up highly dangerous free radicals; it has a particular affinity for one type of particularly dangerous free radical called the hydroxyl radical."[1] He pointed out that, as a result of this phenomenon, salicylic acid is often used as a lab test for hydroxyl radicals.

Instructions for Using Salicylic Acid

When you buy your salicylic acid product, please read the label carefully and choose one with a 2% concentration. A lower percentage may not be effective; more is unnecessary and therefore not worth paying for. Salicyclic acid products come in many forms, all equally effective. Among the best-selling ones with the correct concentration are Zapzyt, PropapH, Stridex, and Oxy Night Watch.

Also, when you purchase a salicylic acid product, make sure that it does not include any other active ingredients, especially glycolic acid. That's the product for Step 2 of the Acne Cure program. In Dr. Dubrow's clinical experience, if you handle the two steps in one application, they tend to interfere with each other and are likely to be less effective than if you apply them separately. We do not fully understand why this is so. Perhaps there is a chemical reaction between the two reagents, rendering each of them less potent. Or perhaps the cleaning ability of one in effect "cleans away" the other. But then there are many mysteries in medicine. Fortunately, we don't have to understand everything about *how* a system works to know that it *does* work.

Whatever product you choose, use it twice daily for the 6 weeks of the program (or until your acne has entirely disappeared) as follows:

1. Wet the skin of the acne-affected area with warm water. (If you have several areas with acne, deal with them one at a time.)

2. Pour a small amount (about the size of a penny) of the salicylic acid lotion into your palm.

3. Add a few drops of water, and rub until the water and lotion are completely mixed.

4. Gently massage the mixture into the skin in a circular motion. Make sure you cover the entire area that has any signs of acne—it's better to cover too much than too little.

5. Repeat the process in the other affected areas—chest, back, and so on. (You'll need to get some help to work on your back if you cannot reach.)

6. Leave the lotion in place for a while (say, for as long as it takes you to brush your teeth), and then rinse off with warm water, possibly by taking a shower.

7. Do this first thing in the morning, for men immediately after you shave, and last thing at night.

STEP 2

REMOVING THE CLOG

The salicylic acid of Step 1 is not designed to remove plugs of sebum and cells that are already clogging pores; rather, its role is to cleanse the surface of the skin of *excess* dry cells and bacteria, not to try to remove *all* dry cells and bacteria. The task of digging down and first loosening and then removing the "cemented-in" plugs calls for sterner stuff, namely glycolic acid.

Glycolic acid is close to a medical miracle. But until recently we had little idea how it works. Even now, its exact mechanisms remain something of a mystery. Part of its action is obvious: It has considerable solvent power and can therefore dissolve any plugs it can reach. But, as we have explained, most of the plugs are inside closed pores and therefore not reachable. Yet glycolic acid manages to loosen and remove many of these too. Only limited research has been conducted on just how glycolic acid performs this additional trick of dissolving plugs beneath the skin's surface. The best information we have suggests it does so in two ways.

Glycolic acid appears to have considerable antioxidant power to help reduce inflammation and swelling. This helps it to open previously closed pores.

Its other—and perhaps more important—characteristic is its ability to activate certain skin enzymes that "dissolve" the blocking plugs beneath the skin's surface, again helping to open up the pores and leach out the pent-up sebum-and-pus mixture they contain.

Even though medical science doesn't understand exactly how glycolic acid works, Dr. Dubrow has seen it work over and over again in patients to whom he has prescribed it to attack surface plugs and penetrate deeper. In fact, he has observed that glycolic acid not only digs down into pores but also has the ability to carry certain other medications down with it.

Glycolic acid is a natural food product derived from sugar cane. It is one of the most popular of the alpha hydroxyl acids—mild, natural, organic acids used in a large number of rejuvenating cosmetic creams. Indeed, it is one of relatively few cosmetic products that are efficacious in removing some of the dead skin cells on the surface of the stratum corneum without excess harshness, giving skin a younger appearance while rarely (at least in low concentrations) doing damage.

Some of the more recognized brands of glycolic acid, which comes in various forms, are Gly Derm, Cellex-C, Total Skin Care, and Physician's Elite. If you have trouble finding the recommended concentration, consult with a skin care specialist.

Instructions for Using Glycolic Acid

When choosing your glycolic acid product, look for one that has between 8 and 10% active ingredient and contains no other active ingredients. (As explained above, one step at a time!)

Apply the glycolic acid cream in the morning after the salicylic acid treatment, using the identical application technique. Leave it on for a few minutes before rinsing it off with warm water. Continue for the whole 6 weeks, or until your acne disappears.

STEP 3

STOPPING THE DISEASE
DEAD IN ITS TRACKS

The first two steps of the program will smooth out the surface of your skin, remove a large number of the cell–sebum wads that were clogging your pores, and eliminate most of the nasty surface bacteria that help perpetuate acne infections. At the same time, they also remove all sorts of other noxious bacteria that could infect your open wounds (which is what acne lesions are).

As if your acne weren't problem enough, secondary bacterial infections can be even worse. Sometimes they can be treated only with antibiotic injections, but as we have noted, this is undesirable unless absolutely necessary.

However, if you limited your efforts to only these two steps, even though those wads have been loosened and, in many cases, washed out, your pores would remain inflamed and hence swollen down their length. Consequently, infected sebum, pus, and *P. acnes* germs would still lurk in the follicular canals—and the farther from the skin's surface, the more virulent they would be. So, unless there is a way to reach into those interstices and clean them out, your acne would soon revive. Indeed, that is exactly what usually happens with the use of commercial acne remedies: Sufferers experience temporary relief but then find that their condition continues or even worsens.

While Dr. Chu, in *The Good Skin Doctor*, and others like him have paid lip service to the view that acne can be treated, the fact that most of the existing cures on the market fail to render long-term relief has prompted them to give away their real belief that acne is largely incurable. Dr. Chu wrote, for example, "Even if you suffer from acne, we believe it's possible to make the most of yourself and look as good as you can."[3] There would be no need for him to make such an exhortation if he were convinced that acne could be permanently eradicated.

The reason our Acne Cure program works is that, in addition to cleaning the surface of the skin with salicylic acid and loosening many of the surface "wads" with glycolic acid, it adds a third vital step.

As we have emphasized before, the single most effective way of destroying the *P. acnes* bacteria within your pores is to douse them with an antibacterial agent. Fortunately, there is such an agent, and a very efficient one. It is called benzoyl peroxide (or BP for short). It undoubtedly works better than any oral or topical antibiotic at killing *P. acnes*. And because it produces oxygen—in the presence of which *P. acnes* do not thrive—the bacteria can never develop immunity to BP.

However, even after the salicylic acid and the glycolic acid have done their work, many of your pores may remain so clogged with the swelling caused by inflammation that the BP (or any other topical medication) can't reach the bacteria hiding deep inside your skin. The solution is a technique widely used by plastic surgeons and dermatologists, though barely known outside those professions. It is to reduce the inflammation and open up the pores by making the skin cold.

We realize that this sounds simplistic and perhaps old-fashioned. But it is the most effective way we've seen to prepare the skin to take in the BP. It works!

Instructions for Using Benzoyl Peroxide (BP)

Here is what to do each evening after you have applied and washed off the salicylic acid.

1. *Run an ice cube over the area you intend to treat to cool down the skin until it is thoroughly wet and feels cold to the touch, but be careful not to freeze your skin.*

2. *Apply the BP (that you have kept cold in your refrigerator) using essentially the same technique you used for the salicylic acid and the glycolic acid. However, first cool the palm of your hand with the ice cube to avoid warming up the BP too much. Place a small amount of the cool BP cream or lotion in your palm, then apply it evenly across all areas of the skin that show any traces of acne.*

3. Once you have applied the BP over the affected (and cool and wet) area, place one or more cold packs on the affected areas. (Obviously, if you suffer from acne front and back, you'll have to handle your problem in two treatments.) Leave the ice packs in place for about 10 minutes while you lie down and relax. You can use the cool packs they sell in most drugstores, keeping them in the freezer until needed; or you can simply wrap up some ice cubes in toweling. Be careful not to freeze your face; just keep it comfortably cold. (If it gets too cold, just put some more towels between the pack and your skin.)

4. When you're through, wipe off any excess BP with a soft, dry cloth, leaving the residue in place to work on bacteria all night.

You will probably feel a slight tingling a short while after you apply the BP. But even if you don't, be certain that the cold has constricted your blood vessels, minimizing the swelling that is clogging your pores. The BP is penetrating deep into those pores. The inflammation is receding. *P. acnes* can run, but now it can't hide!

If you feel more than a comfortable tingling when you use the BP—that is, if you note itching, burning, redness, scaling, or excessive dryness—then start alternating your use of the glycolic acid and BP: one on Monday, the second on Tuesday, and so on. However, in that case, use the cold pack procedure with the glycolic acid as well as with the BP. It's important that you reduce the inflammation and swelling around your pores with the cold pack every day.

The Benefits of Cold

The beauty of this third, vital step in the Acne Cure program is that it kills three birds with one stone:

1. The cold has the effect of opening the pores where the bacteria are hiding, letting the BP do its work.

2. By reducing the inflammation, it reduces the swelling around the pores, and thus it lessens the likelihood of other pores becoming clogged.

3. And 10 minutes under a pleasantly cool face pack is a wonderful relaxant. (Some people enjoy this cold pack routine so much that they continue to use it, without the BP, after their acne is long forgotten.) As we shall discuss in chapter 10, stress of all sorts is well known to aggravate acne. "Spacing out" for 10 minutes at the end of your day while you feel the medicine working to eliminate your acne will relieve a surprising amount of tension.

Since the cold reduces inflammation by constricting the blood vessels so that less blood rushes in and the swelling recedes, the following question might occur to you: Does less blood around the skin mean that fewer of the blood's natural infection fighters, such as white corpuscles, are available to heal your acne lesions? Fortunately the opposite applies.

As you know, many sports injuries are treated with ice packs. The initial impact of the ice is to reduce the inflammation and the resultant swelling by shrinking the blood vessels and, so, slowing down the rush of blood to the area. However, the body also has an opposite reaction to the cold, namely to send extra blood to the chilled area to warm it up. (You may have noticed this phenomenon yourself when you've had very cold hands. As soon as you came inside or otherwise warmed your hands, they seemed to glow.) Fortunately, however, the body sends this warming blood to the area gradually, without causing re-swelling. Thus, the sports physician has given his patient the best of all worlds: reduced swelling and inflammation but increased flow of curative blood.

Similarly, cooling your face first shrinks the blood vessels, opens the pores, and lets the BP in. Then, a short time later, the body sends extra blood to the area to warm it again. It does so gradually and so avoids renewed swelling and inflammation. Nevertheless, that extra influx carries with it extra white corpuscles with their curative impact.

STEP 4

PROTECTING YOUR SKIN

The first three steps of the Acne Cure program will get rid of your acne in all but the most intractable cases within no more than 6 weeks.

The fourth step, which you should start right away and then continue permanently, is to keep your skin healthy, soft, good-looking, and resistant to new attacks. At the minimum, this involves using a moisturizing cream daily. The best time to apply it is after washing the affected area so that you keep in place as much moisture as possible. However, there is more to maintaining great skin than that.

But first, two caveats:

1. Make sure you use an oil-free moisturizer. Oily moisturizers tend to combine with your own sebum to form those undesirable clogs.

2. Always use a moisturizer that contains a sunblock of SPF 15 or higher. Ultraviolet light does skin more harm than all the other insults combined. And the damage it causes increases the cells' slough-off rate and weakens the skin's resistance to bacterial attack—both of which encourage acne formation. In any case, who wants unnecessary wrinkles? And remember, you need the sunblock almost as much when it's cloudy as when the sun is shining. Ultraviolet light is a major component of *all* daylight, not just sunlight. Plants need ultraviolet light to thrive, but they do just fine in England and the Scandinavian countries where it is cloudy for much of the year.

However, using an oil-free moisturizer with a sun block is only Step 4 at its most basic level. In practice, there is a lot more to keeping your skin in immaculate condition. Moreover, if you have suffered from acne for any length of time, you may have been so active in trying to cure yourself that you simply haven't had time to worry about the rest of the problems that can harm your skin, dull your complexion, give you premature wrinkles, or do all of those in combination.

Once your acne is a problem of the past, it is time to move beyond just using a moisturizer. From now on, you should complete the process and make sure your skin looks fully healthy (that is to say, better than just acne-free) and as beautiful and radiant as it deserves to look. That is what chapters 6 and 7 will help you to achieve—now and for a long time to come.

5

THE RESEARCH PROOF

MANY BOOKS ON SKIN CARE—and on other health subjects too—are little more than one person's opinion. At best, they are supported by very little research—and that often conducted by the authors themselves and never published in a peer-reviewed journal where other scientists have the opportunity to criticize or support the research methodology and results.

In this case, however, every aspect of the Acne Cure program Dr. Dubrow developed has been fully researched and the results published in medical journals throughout the world. It is the *combination* of these beneficial products (plus the use of cold to make one of them more effective) that is new—and makes the whole more effective than the sum of its parts.

Thus, for readers who are interested in the research support for the Acne Cure described in the prior chapter, we will summarize a number of the main studies behind each of the three medications that constitute the cure itself: salicylic acid, glycolic acid, and benzoyl peroxide (BP). Then, in the next chapter, we will discuss in more detail (and provide research support for) how to maintain your skin in the best possible condition once your acne is cured.

Virtually every research study we have found on salicylic acid, glycolic acid, and benzoyl peroxide indicates that each of these medications has proven helpful in treating acne but that none is fully curative. That, of course, is why both researchers and acne sufferers conclude that the disease is incurable.

However, we have not been able to unearth a single mention in all the scientific literature that suggests that a combination of these three medications, applied in parallel but separately, would have the effect of almost completely eliminating acne.

Nor is there any mention in the literature of the use of cold to open pores and let the BP in to do its work. There is ample research about the use of cold packs and ice on strains and sprains and bruises. And plastic surgeons frequently utilize cold to reduce the swelling and inflammation in their postoperative patients. But apparently no one has thought of cooling the skin as a way of improving the potency of BP. Yet, as Dr. Dubrow discovered, that is the way the medication works most efficiently (while, concurrently, the other medications make their contributions). With cold having shrunk the swelling of the pores caused by their inflammation, the BP can penetrate to where *P. acnes* hides.

Given the depth of research behind each medication involved in Dr. Dubrow's protocol, coupled with cold's universally accepted ability to reduce inflammation and its resultant swelling, we cannot help but find it surprising—in fact, amazing—that no one else has developed a protocol combining these well-known, scientifically proven ingredients into a single program that effectively eradicates acne.

SALICYLIC ACID

The first step in treating acne is to use a salicylic acid wash. There is ample evidence that salicylic acid is an effective first attack. For example, in 1992, E. Zander and S. Weisman reviewed four studies on the safety and efficacy of 0.5% and 2.0% solutions of salicylic acid.[1] The results from all four studies showed that salicylic acid pads "reduced the number of primary lesions and therefore the number and severity of all lesions associated with acne."

These findings have been widely duplicated. In Richmond, Virginia, B. A. Johnson and J. R. Nunley explained, "Comedonal acne usually responds to . . . salicylic acid."[2] In Czechoslovakia, Z. Fendrich and colleagues (writing in Czech) stated flatly that "salicylic acid . . . when used on the long-term basis . . . reduces the number of microcomedones and counteracts plugging of the follicles."[3] And in 1981, A. R. Shalita, a professor of dermatology at the State University of New York, published the results of a study of 49 patients with mild to moderate acne who used Stridex (a cream containing 0.5% salicylic acid) for a month. He concluded that there was "a significant reduction in inflammatory lesions and open comedones."[4]

However, as we now know, salicylic acid is only a first step. In an earlier test on 30 patients, Dr. Shalita compared a 2% salicylic acid wash with a 10% BP wash.[5] He found two fascinating results. One was that the patients treated with the salicylic acid cleanser showed significant improvement for a while, but by no means a complete cure for their condition. The other finding was that, when the patients switched after 2 weeks to benzoyl peroxide, there was no further improvement. Given what we now know, neither of these results is surprising. The salicylic acid alone could not cure the entire condition because it only attacked one aspect of it. And the BP was relatively ineffective because it was operating on closed pores, where it can do little good.

Even though these and many other studies attested to the efficacy of salicylic acid, some concern grew in the mid-1990s that darker skin might react differently to the medicine due to its higher melanin content. This concern was laid to rest by the 1999 publication of a study conducted by P. E. Grimes, M.D.[6] Dr. Grimes treated 25 dark-skinned patients, who had a variety of acne and acnelike conditions, with high-concentration (20 to 30%) salicylic acid peels, and repeated the procedure five times at 2-week intervals. Even at these very high levels, he found that 88 percent of his patients improved, and only 16 percent had any negative side effects, none more than minimal to mild, and none lasting.

We do not recommend that concentration of salicylic acid since we are using the product as a general cleanser, not a peeling agent. However, the research clearly demonstrates that salicylic acid is safe even on darker skin.

In summary, as the first step in treating acne—but only as a first step—salicylic acid is proven to be safe and effective.

GLYCOLIC ACID

Dermatologists have long used glycolic acid, one of the most widely used of the broadly popular alpha hydroxyl acids (AHAs), as an efficacious chemical peel. Even in strong concentrations, it has few negative side effects, and it creates significant improvements in acne in every type of skin. Thus, it is surely no surprise that, as we described in chapter 4, glycolic acid is an essential part of Dr. Dubrow's Acne Cure program.

As W. P. Smith wrote in the *International Journal of Cosmetic Science*, AHAs "are clearly one of the most exciting cosmetic ingredients used today to combat the visible effects of aging."[7] More recently, R. C. Tung and colleagues agreed that "Acne . . . patients can see improved results when standard regimens are supplemented with AHA peels and lotions."[8] And Eugene J. Van Scott, M.D., of the department of dermatology at the Skin and Cancer Hospital in Philadelphia reported almost 20 years ago that hyperkeratinization—that is, a thickened stratum corneum—is "either a primary or a principal associated event in a majority of dermatological disorders" and that "the therapeutic result of AHAs . . . is not only to improve the skin surface cosmetically but also to improve the flexibility of the stratum corneum" and thus reduce the negative effects of hyperkeratinization.[9]

Among the many studies proving both the efficacy and safety of glycolic acid, one of the more impressive was by a group of three doctors in an Italian university.[10] They conducted glycolic acid peels on 32 cases of normal acne and 40 patients with more severe acne (including eight with cystic acne, which is the toughest of all). They concluded that, in all cases, glycolic acid peels of a 70% concentration induced "rapid improvement and restoration to normal-looking skin." There were virtually no side effects.

In a 1988 12-week, multicenter, double-blind study (that is, one where neither the researcher nor the patient knew which product was being used on each person, thus avoiding any possible researcher bias), M. C. Spellman, M.D., and S. H. Pincus, M.D., compared a combination of two similar acids, azelaic and glycolic, with retinoid, a well-regarded acne medicine.[11] The results favored the azelaic/glycolic acid mixture by a substantial margin.

Similar studies have been conducted on both Asian skin[12] and Black skin.[13] In both cases, the studies—conducted in universities in, respectively, Taiwan and Tunis—showed that glycolic acid, at strengths varying from 15% to 70%, was efficacious in improving acne.

In a thorough study conducted in Turkey, among 58 women, the conclusion was not only that glycolic acid helped cure acne but also that "long-term daily use of low-strength [glycolic acid] products may also have some useful effects on scars."[14]

Again, the effects of glycolic acid are as pronounced in Asian skin as elsewhere. This was proven in a fairly recent study conducted by four physicians in Taiwan.[15] They tested various levels of glycolic acid on 40 Asian patients with "moderate to moderately severe" acne. They found two matters of importance. One was that it took "consistent and repetitive treatment" with glycolic acid to make much difference on cystic acne lesions. This, of course, is hardly surprising since, as we have described, it takes acne some time to "mature" and reach the surface of the skin.

Their more substantive finding—not surprising, either, but reassuring—was that "glycolic acid has considerable therapeutic value for acne with minimal side effects . . . in Asian skin." They concluded with careful scientific reticence that glycolic acid "may be an ideal adjunctive treatment of acne." They are quite right. As we now know, glycolic acid is very effective, but wholly so only when it is used as part of our complete program.

All the research indicates clearly that glycolic acid helps acne. Thus, while it is not itself a cure, it is an integral part of our program.

Moreover, glycolic acid also has other skin benefits that indirectly have a positive effect on the disease: It makes the skin less sensitive to ultraviolet light (thus reducing the impact of photoaging), improves its moisture retention, and, perhaps for the same reasons, improves its general condition.

In two interrelated studies, N. V. Perricone, M.D., and J. C. DiNardo, M.D., concluded that treating sun-burned skin for 7 days with glycolic acid caused a 16 percent reduction in its irritation.[16] They also found that glycolic acid made skin more resistant to attack by sunlight. Specifically, 3 weeks of such treatment gave skin a sun protective factor (SPF) of 2.4. They concluded that glycolic acid was an effective anti-inflammatory and that "the data . . . support the conclusion that glycolic acid acts as an antioxidant."

In a study conducted by Dr. DiNardo (one of the more prolific researchers on glycolic acid) on the effects of various levels of glycolic acid, he and two of his colleagues found that, after 3 weeks of product application (and 1 week off), there was a thickening of the epidermis and "marked increases" in collagen content.[17] They concluded that glycolic acid "demonstrated significant improvement in the condition of the skin."

In a 1996 study of 20 elderly subjects with dry skin, J. C. DiNardo and his colleagues showed that the "water binding properties of the skin were . . . increased by 60 to 70 percent during treatment with 8% glycolic acid."[18]

And in Australia, researchers found that, in a double-blind, clinical study where a 5% glycolic acid cream was compared with a placebo cream, after 3 months of daily use, the patients who had used the glycolic acid cream showed a "statistically significant improvement" versus the control group "in general skin texture and discoloration."[19]

From this body of research, the conclusion is inescapable that glycolic acid, used alone, is fairly effective against acne, and (even at much higher concentrations than we recommend) is safe. By itself, it is not a complete solution, of course. But it plays its essential role as the second step in our four-part Acne Cure.

BENZOYL PEROXIDE (BP)

The third step in the Acne Cure program is benzoyl peroxide. Like the medications involved in the two prior steps, it has been widely researched and proven to be safe and, even on its own, somewhat effective. A. M. Kligman, M.D., Ph.D., is widely recognized as a leading expert on acne. He described BP as an "old warhorse." It has been around since 1905 is used widely to bleach fabrics and flour. It has been sold as an ointment for skin and acne problems since the 1930s, although it was not officially registered for acne treatment until 1960. "It is worth emphasizing," wrote Dr. Kligman, "that benzoyl peroxide depopulates *P. acnes* much faster and to a greater extent than oral antibiotics. Negligible numbers [of the bacteria] are recoverable after 2 weeks."[20]

Many other researchers have echoed Dr. Kligman's favorable view of BP. For example, back in 1980, N. Hjorth of the University of Stockholm wrote that quite a few traditional treatments "make acne worse rather than better. There is evidence that sulphur, soap, and light treatment prolong the course of illness."[21] But, he added, "fortunately, traditional treatment can be abandoned in favor of the superior benzoyl peroxide."

Indeed, the efficacy of BP is so well-established that in recent years most research conducted on it has concentrated on determining whether BP in combination with other acne products can improve the performance of the combination over either agent individually. For example, in 2001, J. J. Leyden, M.D., led a study of 480 patients that compared a combination of 5% BP and clindamycin, a well-established antibiotic, with each of those ingredients separately. The BP–clindamycin combination proved to be more powerful than the BP alone, but each was effective.[22]

Separately, Dr. Leyden conducted a 10-week blind study of 492 patients in which he and his colleagues compared BP alone with BP combined with (a) clindamycin and with (b) erythromycin.[23] The results were impressive: In all three versions, patients showed significant improvements in their inflammatory lesions.

While the combination of BP and clindamycin was the best of the three, the combination of BP and this antibiotic is considerably more expensive than BP alone—and simply not necessary. When BP is used as part of the three-part protocol we have described, it is fully effective in eliminating acne—and once the acne is gone, there is obviously no need for cures that are theoretically more efficacious but practically much more costly.

Moreover, there is another angle to this issue. As shown in a study conducted over a 12-week period by J. J. Leyden, M.D., and S. Levy, M.D., *P. acnes* develops resistance to antibiotics: There is "an increase in the number of resistant bacteria . . . from patients using clindamycin alone, while counts of resistant bacteria remain stable or declined in those using the combination gel [of 5% BP and 1% clindamycin]."[24] On the other hand, *P. acnes* never gets acclimated to BP.

There is no doubt that BP works effectively in fighting acne, and works better than almost anything else (except, of course, a combination of products as we have described). Thus, Dr. Kligman wrote, "No prescription antibiotic can begin to match the antibacterial efficacy of benzoyl peroxide. Twice daily applications for 5 days will reduce the *P. acnes*'s population by more than 95 percent! Neither clindamycin nor erythromycin can match that level after 2 to 3 months. . . . Benzoyl peroxide has to receive high marks for therapeutic performance."[25]

Dr. Kligman is by no means alone in his assessment that BP is "the best there is." For example, V. B. Patel, M.D., found in a study that BP was as effective as topical tretinoin in the "percentage reduction in total number of skin lesions."[26]

There is more good news. As it turns out, BP is not only effective as an acne fighter; it is also a very versatile drug with other significant skin benefits. For, as G. Valacchi, M.D., and colleagues, among others, have tried to explain, besides its antibacterial activity, BP also seems to have an antioxidant impact.[27] Exactly how this works is not fully understood. But for our purposes, suffice it to say that it does.

CONCLUSION

The research proves that by itself, each aspect of the Acne Cure program, developed by Dr. Dubrow and described in chapter 4, is reasonably effective at treating acne without being able to cure it. The *combination* of these medications, coupled with the appropriate use of cold, for the reasons we have described, should logically eliminate the problem entirely in the large majority of patients. To date, there has been no full statistical study to prove that. However, Dr. Dubrow has found that, in almost every case, he has been able to clear up the disease in his patients sometimes within days, nearly always within a few weeks.

So, try it for yourself. You will see your acne disappear.

6

BEAUTIFUL SKIN

ONCE YOUR ACNE HAS BEEN ELIMINATED, your skin—and with it your whole face—will look dramatically better. Gone will be the pimples, black- and whiteheads, blotchy redness, enlarged pores, and occasional scabs. But that is not all: You will have the opportunity of making further improvements in the condition of your skin. With just a minimum of extra effort (probably less than you wasted on unsuccessfully treating your acne before you heard of our cure), you can take a huge step beyond healthy skin, all the way to glowing and radiant skin.

Moreover, by following the correct skin program—for men as well as women—you will be able to maintain young-looking, healthy, vibrant skin throughout your lifetime. By doing so, of course, you will also reduce the likelihood that your acne will ever recur. And, if you are unfortunate enough to be left with scars from earlier acne, you will see them become less visible even before you apply the more vigorous scar reduction techniques we cover in chapter 12.

Madame Helena Rubinstein, one of the founders of the modern cosmetics industry, used to say that there is no such thing as an ugly woman, only a lazy one! And she proved it by developing a series of skin care products that worked remarkably well. Madame Rubinstein believed the same of men. In fact, she was one of the first cosmetic entrepreneurs to develop a skin care line for men. The slogan of the Helena Rubinstein Company in its now-forgotten heyday was "The

Science of Beauty." Even in those days long before today's advanced skin care products were invented, careful skin treatment could do a lot to keep skin young-looking, smooth, and attractive. Today, of course, the science of skin care has advanced tremendously. But the principle still applies: Any man or woman can have young-looking, attractive skin with just a minimum of effort.

Today we know much more than we did in Madame Rubinstein's time about why and how we age, and what we can do about it. It would be an exaggeration to say that men and women can hold aging at bay throughout their lifetime. But we are not exaggerating in the least when we say that most of the wrinkles you see on men and women starting in their thirties and forties—and sometimes even earlier—are unnecessary. In fact, they are largely self-induced.

Not only will a regular, simple skin care regimen stop the reappearance of your acne—or, if it appears, make it so minor that a few days' reversion to the Acne Cure program outlined in chapter 4 will clear it away completely—but it will also give your skin back a natural glow and keep it that way for years to come.

In the opening sentence of his best-selling book *The Wrinkle Cure*, Dr. Perricone stated, "Wrinkled, sagging skin is *not* the inevitable result of growing older. It's a disease, and you can fight it. You can . . . enjoy beautiful skin . . . every day of your life."[1]

A number of the findings in Dr. Perricone's book are controversial, but his central theme, that you do not have to "look your age" when it comes to the appearance of your skin, is not. We wholeheartedly concur.

However, to maintain youthful skin throughout your lifetime, you need to expend a certain amount of effort, and you have to follow a routine. In the balance of this chapter, we will outline the basic steps you need to take to keep your skin in near-perfect condition for the rest of your life. Obviously, if you have already allowed your skin to become wrinkled and old-looking, we cannot guarantee that you will be able to restore it to its full youthful quality. However, even in that case, by following our protocol, you will be able to reduce your wrinkles (even many of those small, hairline wrinkles and tiny lines around your eyes and the corners of your mouth); improve the "glow" of your skin; and enjoy a considerable improvement in the quality and youthful appearance of your skin.

WHAT DAMAGES SKIN?

As we have explained before, by far the largest source of skin damage is ultraviolet light. If you examine a part of your body that is rarely exposed to light—say, your inner thighs—you will see that the skin there looks just about the same as it did when you were a youngster. This applies even to people well into their sixties and beyond. There are no little wrinkles; the skin is still soft and smooth, and its color remains clear and fresh. If you compare that with the skin on your face (assuming you have not been following a skin care protocol that includes an effective sunblock), you will see the difference in an instant.

But the fact is that there is no innate difference between the two areas of skin. The main difference is that one has been exposed to light, while the other has not.

In Bali, where the sun shines almost all the time, it used to be customary for women to spend their lives uncovered from the waist up. Even today, many older Balinese women often go uncovered. Unlike American and European women, whose breast skin, rarely exposed to the sun, is typically smooth and wrinkle-free, Balinese women have chests that look just as wrinkled, leathery, and old as their faces.

The passage of time is not the main reason that your face develops wrinkles. Indeed, wrinkles are unnecessary. We cannot overstress that the main cause of the wrinkles is ultraviolet light—most severely sunlight, but in fact all daylight and even some indoor lights. (Plants cannot live without ultraviolet light. But many green plants live indoors very nicely, including in windowless offices or hospital rooms, where natural light never penetrates. The ultraviolet content of artificial lights, especially fluorescent lighting, is enough to keep them thriving.)

Four different types of rays emanate from the sun. Three of them are forms of ultraviolet light: UVA, UVB, and UVC. The fourth type is infrared light.

UVA Rays

UVA rays are the most abundant and insidious of the sun's ultraviolet rays, present all year round and all day long. They are deceptive because they don't cause sunburn or surface damage to the skin or eyes, but they do penetrate the skin to the dermis (further than any other kind of ray), breaking down and destroying the supporting collagen and elastin fibers. This thins and weakens the dermis, leading to premature aging, wrinkling, and sagging. UVA rays also damage the tiny blood vessels that bring nourishment to the skin, and when those blood vessels are damaged, the skin suffers from a form of malnutrition. This weakened state weakens the body's natural defenses against free radicals; infections, such as acne; cancers; and other diseases.

UVA rays are impressively penetrating. They filter through your closed car window with little loss of potency. And, of course, if you roll your window down, they are joined by the whole spectrum of other rays just waiting to attack the window side of your face and neck, as well as that arm, hand, and thigh. Comparing the left and right forearms of people who drive cars every day and fail to use sunblock on their exposed skin will usually tell the story of considerable sun damage.

UVA radiation damage is cumulative. Signs of damage may not appear for years. But eventually the results of the damage you have done to your skin *throughout your lifetime* will show up as age spots, wrinkles, and sagginess. Even dark-skinned people are susceptible to this kind of damage since melanin filters out little if any of the UVA rays.

UVB Rays

UVB rays are responsible for causing sunburn, freckles, liver spots, and other surface damage to the skin. They are the greatest culprits in causing skin cancers and are responsible for contributing to cataracts and other eye damage. UVB rays are strongest in the summer and between the hours of 10 A.M. and 3 P.M.

UVC Rays

UVC rays are not a problem today because they are blocked out by the ozone layer and do not reach the earth's surface. However the protective layer is developing a hole, which seems to be expanding. It varies in size by season, and its growth is slow, so that it is hard to be sure. However, the evidence is gradually becoming more persuasive. If this continues, then UVC rays will become a problem for which we will have to develop solutions.

No matter where the ultraviolet rays come from, they still damage the skin. Some tanning salons claim that they are "safer than the sun" because they don't contain the burning, UVB rays. While it is true that you do not burn as easily under those circumstances, you do continue to do long-term damage to your skin. These salons are certainly not safe.

Infrared Light

Although infrared light is at the other end of the spectrum from ultraviolet light (that is, its wavelength is just longer than visible red light, whereas UV light's wavelength is just shorter than visible violet light), it too penetrates the skin and is damaging. This is particularly true when it is combined with UVA and UVB rays.

Unfortunately, because it takes years or even decades for the sun-induced damage to appear, many people don't take steps to avoid excessive sunlight until it is too late. In fact, in many cases a significant part of the long-term sun-related skin damage that we see in our forties already occurred by the time we were 20. While some of this damage can be reversed, we would have been better advised to have avoided the damage in the first place.

Other Skin "Wrinklers"

Although ultraviolet light is the worst culprit, there are other causes of wrinkles, too. Chief among them is smoking. As D. J. Leffell, M.D., pointed out in his book *Total Skin*, "the skin of a chronic smoker's face is crosshatched with crevice-like wrinkles and lines often giving the cheeks a tic-tac-toe look."[2] In addition, the constriction in the blood vessels caused by the chemicals in smoke may give the smoker a sallow complexion. In some cases, the skin may even feel cool to the touch, almost clammy.

As anyone who has tried to quit smoking knows, cigarettes are highly addictive, and giving them up is difficult. All we can emphasize here is that you will look younger, healthier, and more vibrant if you do. (You'll also cut down dramatically on your risk of getting lung or other cancers or heart disease . . . but then you knew that!)

Another aging impact on your skin is excess alcohol consumption, that is, more than 2 ounces of alcohol per day. At higher levels than that, you begin to be in danger of generating visible red capillaries on your cheeks and on the end of your nose. Two ounces of alcohol is about the amount in four jiggers of most liquors, four glasses of wine, or four cans of beer. (Of course, the harm alcohol may do depends not only on the quantity you consume but also on the speed at which you consume it. In fact, we would urge you to drink less than 2 ounces daily on a regular basis, and if you do drink that much, never do so at a single sitting.)

Poor skin appearance can be caused by lack of sleep. We have all observed the bags-under-the-eyes, gray look of people who missed their adequate night's sleep. If you have had the experience of taking an overnight, "red eye" flight—say, from California to New York— you may remember that the faces of your copassengers (and, of course, your own face) all seemed "grayed out" as you all stumbled, bleary-eyed, into the airport.

The amount of sleep each of us needs varies. Some people are satisfied with 6 hours a night; others need as much as 8. (However, habitually sleeping more than 8 hours a night may not be good for you. It may even be a sign of depression or of a physical complaint.) However, most people are able to assess for themselves how much sleep they need.

Finally, poor skin appearance can be simply the sign of a poorly balanced diet. We will be talking later about the effect that diet has on skin.

Fortunately, each of these causes is largely within your own ability to control. And, for the most severe of them—namely, sun exposure— the control requires very little effort. All you need to do is to make sure that every morning after you shower or shave, you apply a moisturizer with an SPF rating of at least 15. Unless you plan to spend a lot of time in direct sunlight, that should be sufficient for the day. If you are exposed to lot of sun, you should reapply the moisturizer every few hours.

THE DIFFERENCES IN SKIN

Not all skin is created equal!

The most obvious difference is in the color of your skin. However, those color differences are usually correlated with other differences too. Thus, if you have very white, porcelain skin, you are less likely to suffer from acne—and, if you do, it will generally be less severe. But you are much more likely to suffer from ultraviolet light damage and to develop wrinkles. On the other hand, if you have dark skin, you may have a continuing problem with acne, but you probably won't get crow's-feet or other wrinkles until well past 40 or even into your early fifties. As one of our friends put it, "Black don't crack!"

If you are a typical fair-skinned Nordic type, you are likely to have thin, dry skin that needs to be treated gently. Your best basic skin routine is to use a gentle cleanser, preferably a soap-free, liquid cream cleanser. And then use an oil-free moisturizer (with a sunblock) twice a day or whenever your skin starts to feel dry.

In order to be fully effective, a moisturizer must do three things:

1. It must prevent water from evaporating from the skin.

2. It must allow the skin to continue to "breathe"—that is, take in oxygen and expel carbon dioxide. Using a heavy oil or grease on the skin prevents this process. Thus, a moisturizer should be structured so that its molecules are packed tightly enough to prevent the skin's natural moisture from escaping but loosely enough to allow the skin to breathe.

3. Finally, a good moisturizer should contain one or more humectants, ingredients that attract moisture from the surrounding atmosphere, drawing it into the skin.

Considerable progress has been made in the science that underlies modern moisturizers. For many years, even the best moisturizers could hold water in the skin for only a few hours. In the past few years, however, new moisturizers have been developed that are capable of holding moisture in the skin for much longer. These mois-

---

TRAVEL TIP

Long airplane flights dry out your skin. If you're not careful, you'll arrive a day later, looking a year older! So before a long flight, do something for your skin you wouldn't—and shouldn't—normally do: Give a good covering of a thoroughly oily moisturizer to the skin on your face and anywhere else you may be developing wrinkles—for example, in the upper-chest area just below the chin, where most women's skin—and (in these increasingly tieless times) many men's skin—is regularly exposed to sunlight. Baby oil will do just fine. That will keep the moisture in your skin for the duration of the flight, but you won't keep the oil on long enough to risk acne formation. Then, when you arrive at your destination, clean off the excess oil with your normal gentle cleanser, and remoisturize with your normal, nonoily moisturizer.

---

turizers wash off easily enough, but, if left alone, the best of them will continue to moisturize the skin for remarkably extended time periods—as long as 3 days.

Be especially careful to keep the skin moisturized when you are in a dry atmosphere. Deserts and similar arid locations are obvious examples. Less obviously, the air on very cold, clear days may contain very little moisture and may therefore be desiccating to your skin. When it is cold, air can hold less water vapor than when it is warm (just as cold water will dissolve less sugar than will hot water). But once the dry air filters inside and warms up, it is ready to soak up a lot of extra moisture. And your skin may be an excellent source of that moisture!

Even less obvious is the fact that airplane air is similarly dry. Older people, whose skin already has a tendency to sag and wrinkle, may actually see a temporary increase in wrinkling after a lengthy flight. (Why airplanes don't add a healthy level of humidity to their air supply is a question to which we have no answer!)

If you feel that your whole skin needs moisturizing, here's a tip: Run yourself a warm bath and pour in ½ ounce of baby oil. As you get in and submerge your body, the baby oil will deposit itself uniformly all over your skin. Of course, you can't also wash in the bath, and be careful not to get your hair wet, or it will be full of oil. Also, be careful not to slip as you are getting out of the bath. Both its surface and yours will be slick!

If you are African-American, Hispanic, or Asian, you need a different regimen. We will discuss the specific issues that those of you with ebony to medium brown, brown to olive, and yellow skin face in chapter 9.

Asians tend to be the best off from the point of view of the health of their skin. On the one hand, their skin is less susceptible to sun damage than White skin; on the other, it is also less susceptible to oil, and therefore to acne and keloids, than most Black skin. However, we have found that few advantages in life—and in skin in particular—don't have compensatory disadvantages. The downside of Asian skin is that, when not treated with enough tender loving care, it may start to look sallow, prematurely wrinkled, puffy, and old. The solution is to keep the skin carefully moisturized at all times—and, even more than for other skin types, to get enough sleep.

SPECIFIC SKIN CARE REGIMENS

To be specific, here are the *topical* regimens we urge you to follow, depending on your skin type. (We will discuss later the *internal*, nutritional and antioxidant guidelines that should apply to everyone.)

First, determine whether you have dry, oily, or combination skin. The most usual combination is an oily "T-zone" (that is, the area in the shape of a T comprising your forehead and your nose and often including your chin), combined with dry skin on the rest of your face. If you are not sure what type of skin you have, most of the beauty consultants working in department stores for well-known beauty brands (such as Estée Lauder, Clinique, and Chanel) will be able to tell you. But until you know exactly what you are looking for, resist their attempts to sell you their products.

Once you know what type of skin you have, one of the following protocols will apply to you.

Dry Skin

Make sure to avoid all harsh, oil-dissolving cleansers. Regular soap is not desirable; it does too good a job and, as noted earlier, tends to be alkaline, which is undesirable. Rather, use one of the many mild liquid cleansers formulated for dry skin. If you can find one that contains glycolic acid, that's ideal.

Use plenty of oil-free moisturizer. Reapply several times a day as necessary. And apply a special type of moisturizer (as we discuss below) every night before you go to bed.

Limit your use of makeup, and, when you need it, choose a product formulated for dry skin. You have to select carefully because many of these so-called nourishing foundations contain occlusive oils, which are contraindicated for acne. Try to settle for a product that is not too thick and oily but still adequately moisturizing. (Most cosmetic companies market such compromise products; ask a cosmetician at an established department store for her advice—but there's no need to buy everything she suggests!)

Oily Skin

Contrary to what you may think, it is *not* desirable to use harsh soaps, alcohol-based astringents, or anything else that purports to "dry" excess oil. As we have explained, those products are harmful. There is even some indication that, by drying off the outer sebum, they may stimulate the sebaceous glands to increase the amount of sebum they produce.

However, also avoid "superfatted" soaps, which may actually add oil. Rather, use an oil-binding liquid or a gentle cleanser (preferably with glycolic acid) formulated for oily skin.

Even for oily skin, we recommend the use of a moisturizer—although, obviously, not one with an oil base. Rather, we suggest you use one of several products on the market that are oil-free or water-based. Also, makeup containing glycerin or sodium pyrrolidonecarboxyl acid can be valuable for oily skin since it actually traps water from the surrounding atmosphere and moisturizes the skin without the use of clogging oils. We recommend that you use a moisturizer mornings and evenings.

Finally, for adding color, use powder rather than cream blushes.

Combination Skin

Obviously, you cannot use different treatments on different areas of your face. Thus, the best rule of thumb is to use the skin care products that are suited to the oiliest area. That is where acne is most likely to break out. Moreover, now that you have sworn off the use of harsh or abrasive cleansers and alcohol-based astringents even for the oiliest skin, you will do the dry skin areas of your face no harm by using your oily-skin regimen on them. If that leaves the dry areas a little too dry, just apply a little more moisturizer.

ANTIOXIDANT THERAPY

As we have emphasized, antioxidants, applied topically and taken internally, are vital to the maintenance of all aspects of our health. In a lengthy and erudite summary article, M. P. Lupo covered the large body of research on topical antioxidants. "Since the late 1980s," she wrote, "consumer demand for more effective products . . . has resulted in increased basic science research and product development. . . . The result has been more ingredients that may actually improve not just the appearance of the skin, but the health of the skin as well. We now have products that renew, restore, and rejuvenate—not just cleanse, protect, and moisturize. . . . There are considerable data to suggest the benefits of such ingredients."[3] She then discussed the main cosmetic ingredients that are helpful to skin. These products, which we describe below, are not essential to eradicate acne—Dr. Dubrow's Acne Cure program will do that effectively. However, they may speed up the process, help in the 5 percent of "intractable" acnes that require more vigorous action, and generally help keep your skin healthy and vibrant.

In the balance of this chapter, we will summarize our recommendations on how you can optimize your antioxidant *topical* skin protection. Then, in chapter 7, we will expand on this information by describing what *internal* antioxidants you can ingest, in the forms of nutritional supplements and food, in order to maximize the health of your skin and indeed of your whole body.

The three most powerful antioxidants when it comes to topical skin care are a variation of vitamin C (a widely touted vitamin that is less effective in its normal form because it is not fat soluble) called vitamin C ester; a relatively new derivative of vitamin E (a vitamin that, in its regular form, has been used in skin creams for years with limited effect) called tocotrienol, which is much more effective as an antioxidant than vitamin E itself; and alpha lipoic acid.

In addition, some forms of vitamin B may have significant antioxidant benefits, and two minerals—zinc and selenium—have been proven to be powerful antioxidants and may even be helpful in inhibiting or reducing acne.

Finally, we shall also discuss vitamin A and its derivative, Retin-A. This product, which is not an antioxidant, has been widely researched and proven to be helpful in maintaining healthy skin. It may also help in cases of intractable acne.

Let us discuss first each of these vitamins (in alphabetical order since they are all important), and then the minerals, starting with the most important ones.

Alpha Lipoic Acid

Researchers discovered alpha lipoic acid in 1951. They found that it is an essential component in the energy-producing part of our cells. Later researchers—notably L. Packer, Ph.D., working at the University of California, Berkeley—showed that it is the most important of the three main skin antioxidants both because it is effective in its own right and because it seems to extend the staying power of both vitamin C ester and tocotrienol.[4] At the same time, as noted previously, it is an anti-inflammatory and helps to shrink the swelling of the pores that is contributing factor to the formation of acne.

An exceedingly complicated organ, skin may react in different ways to the same reagents, depending on how those reagents are activated. A case in point: Certain molecules inside our cells, called transcription factors, are usually inert, but when activated by ultraviolet light can induce cells to produce enzymes that harm collagen and ultimately give rise to wrinkling.[5] However, it appears that, in the presence of alpha lipoic acid, this transcription factor sends a different message. Instead of harming collagen, it seems to cause the skin cells to generate a variation of the collagen-destroying enzyme. This variant attacks only already damaged collagen and, in doing so, leaves room for new collagen—and for a reduction in the formation of wrinkles. In some cases, it also causes a notable reduction in already formed wrinkles.

Vitamin A and Its Derivatives

There are several vitamin A derivatives that find their way into cosmetic creams. The most common is retinyl palmitate. Most researchers feel that this vitamin A derivative is relatively ineffective.

On the other hand, nearly every researcher agrees that there is another derivative of vitamin A that is very valuable for skin care—namely tretinoin, better known as Retin-A.

Retin-A is a prescription product based on vitamin A. It strips excess dead cells from the outer layers of the stratum corneum. The reason it is a prescription product and not available over the counter is that it can irritate the skin of certain people, and it can cause discoloration in Black skin. Some physicians also feel that it should not be used during pregnancy or while breast-feeding (although others feel there is no harm in doing so).

While Retin-A should be used conservatively, it is the only product, prescription or otherwise, known to stimulate collagen production. Thus, in addition to stripping the skin temporarily (an effect that wears off once the skin has passed through one or two replacement cycles), it actually encourages the skin to renew itself—and thus causes a meaningful (and sometimes impressive), lasting improvement in the appearance and apparent age of the skin.

A considerable body of research shows that Retin-A repairs UV damage[6,7,8], stimulates collagen production[9], and helps minimize liver spots.[10]

R. Kotrajaras, working with A. M. Kligman at the University of Pennsylvania, tested 61 Thai people for a year with the daily application of 0.05% tretinoin cream and concluded that "after 12 months, a thin band of new collagen was deposited below the epidermis . . . [and] most subjects experienced at least moderate improvement in appearance."[11] In a similar vein, B. A. Gilchrest of Boston University wrote a thorough review paper in which he concluded that "changes in the epidermis and dermis noted after 12 months suggest tretinoin repairs photodamage."[12]

There is no doubt that Retin-A has a beneficial impact on acne, in that it strips the skin, removing some of the surface comedones. However, using Retin-A is not a necessary part of the Acne Cure's basic program. And if simpler, cheaper means can solve the problem, why use more complicated and expensive ones? Nevertheless, as we will see later, it may be a helpful addition in the few cases where our program is not wholly successful.

In summary, we believe that occasional Retin-A treatments under a doctor's supervision are good for your skin. They will help reduce wrinkling and make your skin look healthier. Generally, however, Retin-A is not needed for the treatment of acne.

Vitamin B Complex

These vitamins, found in whole grains and leafy vegetables, have all sorts of uses. For example, vitamin B_5 is often used as a humectant— that is, it is used to hold water in the stratum corneum, thereby softening the skin.

Niacin (vitamin B_3) has an anti-inflammatory impact on the skin and has been shown to improve acne to some extent.[13]

Vitamin C

Vitamin C has long been recognized as one of the most powerful nutritional supplements. Nobel Prize-winner Linus Pauling was convinced that, in large doses, it powerfully strengthened the immune system. Indeed, there are mountains of research attributing all sorts of benefits to vitamin C. It seems to help the production of neurotransmitters in the brain (essential to our ability to think and remember); build up our supply of L-carnitine, one of the major players in converting fat to energy; and aid in the generation of a variety of chemicals that help ward off heart disease and other aging illnesses.

Vitamin C, applied topically, has the ability to quench ultraviolet-induced free radicals. The result can be a significant improvement in the age appearance of skin. For example, in one recent

JAMES LIND: A TREATISE OF THE SCURVY, 1753

A deficiency in vitamin C leads to scurvy—a problem that was already known to ancient Egyptian seafarers in 1550 B.C. and continued to beset all navies until James Lind, a British sea surgeon, published *A Treatise of the Scurvy* in 1753 in which he explained . . .

On the 20th May, 1747, I took twelve patients in the scurvy onboard the *Salsbury* at sea. . . . They all in general had putrid gums, the spots and lassitude, with weakness of their knees. They lay together . . . and had one diet in common to all, viz. water gruel sweetened with sugar in the morning; fresh mutton broth often times for dinner; at other times puddings, boiled biscuit with sugar, etc; and for supper barley, raisins, rice and currants, sago and wine. . . . Two of [the patients] were ordered each a quart of cyder a day. Two others took . . . elixir vitriol three times a day. . . . Two others took two spoonfuls of vinegar three times a day. . . . Two of the worst patients . . . drank half a pint [of sea water] every day. . . . Two others had two oranges and one lemon given them every day. . . . The two remaining patients took [a drink] . . . three times a day of garlic, mustard seed, *rad. raphan*, balsam of Peru and gum myrrh . . . [and] were gently purged three or four times.

The consequence was that the most sudden and visible good effects were perceived from the use of the oranges and lemons; one of those who had taken them, being at the end of six days, fit for duty. The . . . other was the best recovered of any.

12-week double-blind study, 10 patients applied a vitamin C complex to half of their faces, and an inactive cream to the other sides. Of course, they had no idea which cream was which. At the end of the 12 weeks (and twice during the study), independent evaluators compared the two face sides. Once all the results were tabulated, the conclusion was that "a statistically significant improvement of the vitamin C–treated side was seen in the decreased photoaging scores."[14]

Vitamin C has a number of characteristics that came to light during research on asthma patients. Physicians found that large doses of the vitamin inhibited the formation of arachidonic acid or broke it down chemically into a number of harmless substances. Since arachidonic acid is a major agent in the inflammation of living tissue, it is a bad player in aggravating asthma. Not surprisingly, vitamin C also inhibits arachidonic acid in the skin, and thus reduces the inflammation and consequent swelling of the pores.

The problem is that vitamin C applied directly to the skin does little good. It is not fat soluble and therefore cannot penetrate through the oily sebum and into the fat-encircled cells of which skin is constituted.

However, it turns out that vitamin C ester (chemically, ascorbyl palmitate) has all the antioxidant and anti-inflammatory qualities of vitamin C but is also oil soluble. As a result, it can penetrate into the skin, get to work where it is needed, and so perform wonders in keeping the skin wrinkle-free—and, into the bargain, help to inhibit the return of acne.

Vitamin C ester may also stimulate the growth of fibroblasts, which, as described in chapter 1, are vital to the production of collagen and elastin. If this proves to be so, vitamin C ester will go even further than we now realize in repairing damage from scarring and keeping the skin youthful.

Vitamin E

There is a widely held conviction that vitamin E, applied topically, can assist wound healing and reduce scars. According to most experts, this is a deep-rooted consumer conviction that has no foundation in fact—a classic old wives' tale. That is our view too. Moreover, used excessively, vitamin E may cause an allergic reaction in a small number of people. And there is even research conducted by L. S. Bauman and J. Spencer at the University of Miami that concluded, "Topical vitamin E either had no effect on, or actually worsened the cosmetic appearance of, scars. Of the patients studied, 33 percent developed a contact dermatitis."[15]

As it turns out, however, as with so many old wives' tales, this one, while incorrect, is not far removed from the truth. That is because, although vitamin E itself has no measurable effect on healing scars, a component of it, when isolated and applied to the skin, does have considerable anti-aging and possibly even scar curative powers. Initially, cosmetic scientists assumed that the most effective component of vitamin E was tocopherol and its various derivatives. They therefore formulated any number of cosmetic creams that contained these ingredients. Moreover, there was enough research to support the contention that these products were beneficial for the skin for M. P. Lupo to conclude in her summary article that "all this data validates the popularity of vitamin E and its derivatives as antioxidant, rejuvenating ingredients in cosmetics."[16]

More recently, however, scientists have been researching another form of vitamin E, called tocotrienol. Several new products are now being launched containing this ingredient, usually designated as "high potency E," or "HPE" for short.

There is evidence that HPE, when ingested, has powerful antioxidant characteristics. To date, there is little evidence that it can similarly impart antioxidant power to the skin. All we can say at present is that the signs are hopeful and that you would be well-advised to try the product for yourself and see how it works for you.

Zinc and Selenium

Zinc and selenium both have substantial anti-acne powers. While they may not be needed for most patients applying Dr. Dubrow's Acne Cure program, they can do no harm, and they are likely to improve the general condition of your skin—and possibly other aspects of your health. Thus, we recommend their use as part of an overall health program.

G. Michaelsson, M.D., conducted a definitive study on oral zinc in Sweden in 1977. He compared the effects of oral zinc with tetracycline in 37 patients with moderate and severe acne and scored them at the end of the study on the severity of any acne that remained. So effective was the zinc that "no difference in effect between the treatments was seen. After 12 weeks of treatment, the average decrease in the acne score (i.e., in the severity of the acne as measured by independent evaluators) was about 70 percent in both groups."[17] This is clearly an astonishing result. It confirms earlier research by Michaelsson in which, in a 4-week double-blind study, he compared treatment with zinc ointment with both a vitamin A ointment and a placebo. Here too the zinc ointment performed impressively.[18]

G. Michaelsson also studied the effects of selenium. In a study conducted on 42 young men and 46 young women—all between the ages of 13 and 25 and all suffering from fairly severe acne—he found that the male patients receiving selenium had significantly less acne than the control group, who received a placebo without selenium.[19] The results for his female subjects were more difficult to measure because of the interference of birth control pills. However, the researchers reached the conclusion that "a good response was observed, especially in some patients with pustular acne."

THE ACNE CURE BEAUTIFUL-SKIN MAINTENANCE PROGRAM

Many books on skin care overstate the degree to which skin aging can be slowed, overcome, and even reversed. In particular, the claim that you can entirely eliminate the tendency for older skin—and musculature—to sag and "look its age" is, in our view, to exaggerate the state of our remedial abilities.

However, there is no doubt that a great deal can be done to maintain and improve the condition of your skin—and, in so doing, avoid the recurrence of acne.

In summary, we recommend the following four-part, long-term topical skin care:

Step 1: Moisturize

This is really two steps in one: The moisturizer you use should contain the sunblock. Thus, this is only one easy step, even though it has two solid skin care benefits.

1. Avoid the damaging effect of ultraviolet light by using a sunblock every day—and renewing it twice or more during the day if you are in bright sunlight.

2. Moisturize your skin every morning, and repeat during the day if your skin starts to feel dry.

Step 2: Cleanse Mildly

Use a cleanser that contains glycolic acid if you can find one. If you cannot find such a cleanser, then once a week, after cleansing and before applying your regular daytime moisturizer, apply a small amount of glycolic acid cream to the areas that used to suffer from acne.

Step 3: Use Antioxidants

Every day at bedtime, use a cream that contains the antioxidants vitamin C ester, tocotrienol, and alpha lipoic acid. If you can find a product that contains all three, that's ideal. If not, don't worry; just use three different creams and rotate them using one every third night. Make sure the creams are non-oil-based. Again, this step has a double advantage: It moisturizes and antioxidizes your skin at the same time.

Step 4: Try Retin-A

If your doctor agrees to write you the necessary prescription, enjoy a Retin-A treatment occasionally. When you do, follow these simple steps:

1. *Wash your face at night with a gentle cleanser. If your skin is not particularly dirty, simple water will often do.*

2. *Gently massage in a small amount of Retin-A to each of the major planes of your face (forehead, cheeks, chin, and so on).*

3. *Carefully rub in a tiny amount of Retin-A around your eyes, making sure to keep the product out of your eyes.*

4. *When you have finished, get a good night's sleep! In the morning, be particularly sure that you do not forget to put on your sunblock. Now that you have removed part of the stratum corneum, your skin is even more vulnerable to ultraviolet light than usual.*

There, that's all there is to our simple, four-step, beautiful-skin maintenance program. If you follow this protocol, you can be assured of three benefits:

1. Your acne will probably never recur. Even if it does, it will be mild and easily cured if you revert to the full Acne Cure for just a few days.

2. The surface of your skin will hardly age at all from this day forth, and if you already have wrinkles, chances are they will be considerably reduced.

3. The third benefit is more subtle . . . but perhaps even more important than the first two. Because you can now be sure that your pimples won't interfere with your life, and because you will know that your skin looks younger and healthier than it has in years, you will obviously feel better about yourself. You will enjoy renewed confidence, renewed zest, and a renewal in what the French call *joie de vivre*.

7

TAKING CARE OF YOUR SKIN
FROM THE INSIDE

"DIET RICH IN VITAMINS C AND E may pare Alzheimer's risk," the headline in the *Washington Post* blazoned.[1] The *Post*'s journalist was referring to a June 27, 2002, article in the *Journal of the American Medical Association* that summarized two studies, one a Dutch investigation of 5,394 Rotterdam residents, the other involving 815 participants in Chicago.[2] The studies strongly suggested that vitamins C and E, both powerful antioxidants, could help in this most intractable of diseases.

If antioxidants can help Alzheimer's, it is hardly surprising that they can also help improve the condition of your skin and, in doing so, reduce the severity and inhibit the recurrence of acne. While such internal treatments are not essential in most cases of acne (since our Acne Cure protocol takes care of them completely), we judge that the ingestion of antioxidants is likely to reduce the already small incidence of intractable acnes, and thus reduce the need to take such serious, side effect–prone drugs as Accutane.

We have already seen, in chapter 6, that antioxidants applied topically can improve the appearance of aging skin, slow or stop further deterioration, reduce wrinkles, and to some extent improve acne. In this chapter, we will describe how ingesting various vitamins and minerals can help (largely, although not exclusively, through their antioxidant power) keep your skin young, healthy, and acne resistant. At the end of the chapter, we will summarize our recommendation of the "prescription" of vitamins and minerals you should be taking regularly.

The two studies described in the *Washington Post* were doubly interesting because they also suggested that the effectiveness of these vitamins was considerably greater when they were eaten as part of a regular diet than when they were taken as compensatory supplements for a diet inadequate in these vitamins.

The authors of the article were quick to assure people who are taking vitamin supplements that they should continue to do so. However, they also felt that, whenever possible, vitamins should be included as part of a regular diet. In holding the view that naturally ingested vitamins are better than manufactured supplements—but that supplements are still better than nothing—they fell in line with most of the more advanced thinking in the medical community. Thus, for each vitamin or mineral we recommend, we shall also list the foods that are high in that particular nutritional ingredient. We suggest that, wherever possible, you incorporate enough of these foods into your diet to make sure that you are getting essentially all the vitamins and minerals you need. Thus, the supplements (which we also recommend you take regularly) become just that: *supplements* to make sure your diet does not let you even occasionally fall short of vital ingredients.

Part of the reason you need vitamins even if you are eating plenty of the vitamin-rich foods we recommend is that, in the cooking process, many vitamins may be destroyed. In general, boiling degrades vitamins, as does the passage of time. A frozen fruit salad will taste fresh when you thaw it out 6 weeks after freezing it. But it will have little vitamin C left.

In general, therefore, we recommend that you eat as many of the vitamin-containing fruits and vegetables either raw or only lightly cooked.

WHAT ABOUT DIETING?

One of the problems with most health books (whether they are about your health generally or, like this one, about a specific condition) is that they recommend eating programs that are so draconian they would make the ascetic Saint Francis of Assisi wince.

Many health books recommend a diet of 1 tablespoon of olive oil, 4 ounces of fish, and a whole bunch of fresh vegetables *every day*! Oh, and why not have half a scrumptious orange instead of a doughnut as a snack? Then you can nibble on a carrot at the movies, instead of popcorn.

We have a different view. Sure, you want to be healthy and have glowing, acne-free skin. But you shouldn't have to live a life of obsessive and unrelenting "cuisinal" abstinence to achieve it. Fortunately, you don't.

Brenda Adderly, coauthor of this book, recently spent a year living in France. There she noted for herself what has frequently been written about—namely that while French people generally eat exceedingly well, they are rarely obese.

The fact is, as the French keep proving, that you can eat reasonably lavishly and still hold your weight down, do wonders for your skin, and keep yourself healthy until well into old age. You can do this by eating enough but not stuffing yourself at each meal, eschewing snacks between meals, cutting out high-sugar drinks, and, insofar as you possibly can, replacing deep-fried foods (french fries, doughnuts, fried chicken, and so on) with the same foods boiled, broiled, baked, or eaten fresh. If you can also bring yourself to replace your beer and liquor consumption with red wine (another French habit), that will be a bonus.

If you do this, and include the types of vitamin-containing foods we list below—plus take the supplements we recommend every day—you will be living a healthy lifestyle, and doing so without feeling in the least deprived. Rather, you will have more energy, you will feel more alive, your skin will be radiant, your acne won't bother you, and people will complement you on looking rested, relaxed, and years younger.

EFFICACIOUS VITAMINS

The most important vitamins to ingest for the health of your skin are the antioxidants vitamin C, vitamin E, and alpha lipoic acid. In addition, we think a number of other antioxidants and several other essential minerals are important. So let us now look at the nutritional ingredients we recommend, explain what they do in your body, inform you about the foods that contain them, and recommend the daily supplemental dosage you should take for optimal skin and overall health.

Vitamin C

Perhaps the most important of all vitamins is vitamin C. Fortunately, it is easy enough to consume in its natural form. Just drink fresh orange juice—or eat fresh oranges (or pineapples, lemons, or most other fruits, from strawberries to persimmons, as well as tomatoes, broccoli, and most green leafy vegetables).

Unlike the topical application, which calls for vitamin C ester, for internal consumption standard vitamin C is a first-class antioxidant and essential for your health. That is why, as we described earlier, it quickly cures scurvy. Vitamin C works in a number of different ways, not all of which are yet fully understood. However, many are. Thus we know that vitamin C:

• Strengthens (and perhaps increases the number of) our white blood cells, our first line of defense against bacterial and viral infections. As such, it plays a major role in strengthening the immune system. An increasing number of researchers feel that it may therefore play an important defensive role against various cancers (including skin cancer), though the jury is still out on this. Many now agree with Dr. Linus Pauling, who, in addition to winning the Nobel Prize for a different branch of chemistry, also did the original research that led him to conclude that vitamin C helps protect against the flu virus.

• Aids the body in producing L-carnitine, a cellular ingredient that helps convert fat to energy.

• Seems to play an important role in producing the neurotransmitters that carry the electrical currents in our brains—the process that lets us think and remember.

• Helps repair damaged tissue and heal wounds and broken bones. This characteristic of vitamin C limits the damage done to skin by ultraviolet light.

• Is essential to the production of collagen.

By doing as every mother has probably told every child—namely eating all your fruits and vegetables (but, unlike some mothers, not overcooking them)—you should be getting as much vitamin C as you need. However, since this vitamin is water soluble, it washes out of the system rapidly, and you need to replenish your supply daily.

To be on the safe side, we recommend you take a minimum of 1,000 milligrams daily if you are in your twenties or thirties and, after that, gradually increase until, by the time you are in your fifties, you are taking a sustaining level of 5,000 milligrams daily.

If you are already over 50 and have not been taking vitamin C, start gradually and work your way up to the full dosage over a couple of weeks. (A sudden large increase in your vitamin C intake may give you a little gastric discomfort.)

Whatever is the full dosage for your age cohort, take a third of that daily amount about half an hour before breakfast, lunch, and dinner.

Alpha Lipoic Acid

As we have already discussed, this is arguably the most effective antioxidant of all when applied topically. It is similarly effective when ingested. Alpha lipoic acid is believed to reduce inflammatory reactions throughout the body and possibly slow the onset of heart disease and certain forms of inflammatory arthritis.

Moreover, in addition to all its advantages as an antioxidant, alpha lipoic acid also helps to prevent glycation of collagen, the process by which collagen degrades as a result of excess undigested sugar. This property of alpha lipoic acid is particularly valuable to diabetics.

Alpha lipoic acid is available in a number of foods, but not in sufficient quantities to provide the amount your body needs. That is one of the reasons that free radicals do so much damage in our modern world.

We recommend 100 milligrams a day for everyone, but especially for anyone over 40.

Vitamin B Complex

The six most important variations of vitamin B are vitamin B_1, called thiamin; vitamin B_2, riboflavin; vitamin B_5, pantothenic acid; vitamin B_6, pyridoxine; vitamin B_{12}; and folic acid. Taken together—and including some additional B vitamins—these are known as vitamin B complex.

Each of these vitamins has a separate purpose, but they also tend to synergize with one another, reinforcing their individual performance. Taken together (as we recommend), they provide a long list of health benefits, including:

- Transforming carbohydrates into energy

- Improving memory and brain functions

- Boosting energy

- Improving metabolism

- Aiding the immune system

- And, most important for the purpose of preventing the recurrence of acne, promoting and retaining healthy skin.

B_6 is the most important of the B vitamins for skin care since it helps to convert the essential fatty acids in your body into anti-inflammatory substances called prostaglandins. Perhaps even more important to your overall health, it holds in check your homocysteine levels that, if excessive, may contribute to heart disease.

Folic acid is possibly the most widely recognized of the B vitamins among the general public because it helps women produce healthy babies by regulating embryonic and fetal nerve cell formation. Therefore, pregnant women may wish to take additional folic acid, being sure to check with their obstetricians first.

All the B vitamins occur naturally in a wide range of foods, including almonds, avocados, bananas, black beans, brown rice, chicken, corn, eggs, fish (particularly salmon), green leafy vegetables, ham, liver, milk, mushrooms, and yogurt. Many kinds of beans—including soy, peas, lima beans, and lentils—are particularly high in folic acid. However, we estimate that only about 25 percent of the folic acid in food is available to the body. That is partly due to its chemical makeup and partly to the way we cook and process foods.

B vitamins, like C, are water soluble and therefore easily leach out of the body. Thus, they must be consumed daily. We recommend 100 milligrams of B complex daily. We suggest you do not exceed this dose because, while B vitamins are not dangerous, large quantities have been associated with nerve damage.

Vitamin E in the Form of Tocotrienol

As we discussed earlier, the tocotrienol form of vitamin E (called HPE) is an effective antioxidant when applied topically. However, when ingested, vitamin E is also valuable both as tocotrienol and in its traditional form. While both E and HPE are effective, we recommend HPE as probably having the greater impact. Usually, the tocotrienol/HPE you can buy is combined with gamma tocopherol, another form of vitamin E. This is probably desirable since the two together seem to create the maximum antioxidant effect.

Vitamin E is effective in a wide variety of ways, including helping to:

- Repair skin damage

- Protect your heart and circulatory system because it inhibits LDL (the "bad" cholesterol) from clogging up your arteries

- Reduce many other negative effects of free radicals.

In particular there is a continuing conviction among consumers (unsupported by research but so widely observed that it may have some validity) that vitamin E speeds recovery from external wounds and helps to erase scars and stretch marks.

Wheat germ is probably the best source for gamma tocopherol, and rice bran provides the most tocotrienol. However, since you are hardly likely to consume large quantities of these foods, the following foods contain reasonable amounts of vitamin E: most nuts, especially almonds; avocados and mangoes; peanuts and peanut butter; sunflower oil or seeds; and asparagus. However, you are unlikely to get as much of this vitamin as you need from these products. Therefore, we recommend that young people should take 200 IU (international units) a day, with dosages increasing gradually for older people, topping out at 800 IU daily for people 50 or older.

L-CARNITINE

This supplement appears to help repair damaged skin. Thus, it is helpful both to older people seeking to repair sun damage and to younger people aiming to repair damage from acne. We recommend a daily dose of 1,000 milligrams.

MINERALS

There are several minerals that are important for skin health. They are, in the approximate order of their importance, the following.

Calcium

Although we hear much about the benefits of calcium, according to experts it is one of the most deficient minerals in Americans' diets. An estimated 25 million postmenopausal women suffer from osteoporosis—that is, thin and frail bones—because of insufficient calcium intake earlier in their lives.

In addition, calcium is essential in the bloodstream to:

- Regulate heartbeat and maintain healthy blood pressure

- Assist in blood clotting

(continued on page 108)

L-CARNITINE, THE INDISPENSABLE
ESSENTIAL AMINO ACID

Carnitine is actually the result of the combination of two essential amino acids. The term *essential* means we need them to survive but can get them only from foods or supplements because the body does not itself manufacture them. In her book *The Complete Guide to Nutritional Supplements*, Brenda Adderly described these amino acids as follows:

Take away our bones and teeth, and what's left? Amino acids (or proteins) in varying combinations. Amino acids are the raw materials used to build our cells and are necessary for life because they regulate our biologic processes by creating enzymes, hormones, and neurotransmitters. The 22 amino acids come from our food and, in turn, combine to create over 50,000 different protein molecules that are vital for our bodies to function.

Eight of the amino acids are essential. . . . The remaining 14, though equally vital for life, can be made from the essential eight. The essential aminos are isoleucine, leucine, lysine, methionine, phenylalanine, threonine, tryptophan, and valine. The nonessential aminos are: alanine, asparagine, aspartic acid, cysteine, glutamic acid, glutamine, glycine, proline, serine, and tyrosine. Four other nonessential aminos—arginine, carnitine, histadine, and taurine—are particularly important for infants and children. In fact, children require higher quantities of protein-rich foods per pound of body weight than adults do.

We get amino acids from our diet. "Complete" proteins are in animal foods such as eggs, meat, fish, and milk. They're complete because they contain all eight of the essential aminos. "Incomplete" proteins are found in plant foods and contain fewer than the essential eight. Plant proteins can be combined, however, to provide the essential aminos needed for optimal health. The National Institutes of Health suggest that, for this purpose, good plant proteins include legumes, soy products, and whole grains. Because running on less than the eight essentials can keep the ones we do have from functioning properly, it's important to get them all into our diets. Amino acids require vitamins B_6, B_{12}, and niacin in order to be metabolized, so be sure to include these vitamins when taking supplements. Also, look for supplemental formulas that mirror real proteins so that the much-needed balance of essential and nonessential amino acids— and their correct proportions—are included.

In 1625, Francis Bacon, the great English philosopher who once boasted, "I have taken all knowledge to be my province," wrote: "There is a wisdom in this beyond the rules of physic. A man's own observation, what he finds good of and what he finds hurt of, is the best physic to preserve health." We agree. To remain healthy, protect your skin, and limit your vulnerability to acne, you should not try to adhere to a draconian diet, or deny yourself the foods you love. Rather, you should eat in moderation, follow the supplements program we have suggested, and enjoy yourself!

• Transmit the electrical impulses that make our muscles contract and thus, among other things, limit the "sag" of older faces.

The main source of dietary calcium is milk. One reason that this country faces a calcium deficiency is that people on low-calorie diets often cut out all dairy products. Ironically, fat-free milk, a legitimate part of most diets, contains just as much calcium as whole milk. You can also find calcium in beans, nuts, tofu, and chickpeas. Certain vegetables are also calcium rich, including spinach, broccoli, kale, and potatoes.

Even if you consume reasonable quantities of calcium-containing foods, you are not likely to get as much calcium as your body needs. We therefore recommend that you take 1,000 milligrams daily. But remember to drink plenty of water since calcium may otherwise be somewhat constipating.

Magnesium

Magnesium helps in strengthening bones and in tuning up the cardiovascular system. It does this, in conjunction with calcium, by building up the blood vessels so that they are flexible and strong. It also helps muscles relax. For example, it is helpful in people who suffer from muscle cramps.

Women suffering from premenstrual syndrome and its accompanying headaches, sore breasts, and depressed moods often find relief from magnesium.

If you live in a "hard"-water area, you can get considerable quantities of magnesium from water. Food sources include many types of seafood, particularly flounder, and also milk, cheese, and most nuts and beans. Bananas are a good source of magnesium; many athletes swear that a single banana will cure even the worst sports-induced muscle cramp.

We recommend 200 milligrams daily. However, with your doctor's advice, you may want to double that if you are over 50.

Chromium

Chromium has developed a strong and justified reputation as a fat burner, an effect it achieves by increasing muscle tissue at the expense of fat. More important, researchers have found that chromium is an essential mineral for producing insulin, the hormone that controls the level of sugar in the blood. When the pancreas produces insulin appropriately, a task in which it is aided by an adequate level of chromium, the insulin keeps people from the extremes of too much blood sugar (diabetes) or too little (hypoglycemia).

Beer drinkers will be happy to know that their favorite beverage is a good source of chromium, thanks to the brewer's yeast it contains. However, beer is also a major source of calories, and is therefore likely to result in your weight rising to unhealthy levels, as evidenced by the "beer belly" typical of heavy beer drinkers. You can take chromium from other foods, including beef, cheese, chicken, clams, liver, broccoli, grape juice, and whole grain breads. (Note that grain loses about three-quarters of its chromium content when it is refined.)

We recommend 200 micrograms daily.

Selenium

Selenium is a highly effective antioxidant. It is a trace mineral found in most soils and absorbed by many of the vegetables we eat. Most important, selenium is an essential ingredient of glutathione peroxidase, one of the most potent antioxidants at work in our bodies. This chemical boosts the immune system and (although the research on this is still inconclusive) may help to prevent some cancers.

Selenium works most effectively in combination with vitamins A and E, with the three substances enhancing one another's performance.

Broccoli, garlic, onions, red grapes, as well as oatmeal, brown rice, and other whole grains, may be rich in selenium. However, this is something of a gamble because large tracts of American farmlands appear to have been stripped of selenium, leaving the foods grown there deficient in this essential mineral. In addition, cooking robs most foods of selenium, as does cooking foods. In this instance, supplementation is essential.

We recommend 200 micrograms daily.

Zinc

Zinc is a remarkable mineral. Among its other benefits, zinc contributes to wound healing and, as a separate function, helps maintain sufficient collagen. In some cases, it seems to encourage the healing of acne scars. Obviously, in all three of these respects, it is beneficial to the skin.

Zinc also has many other health benefits For one thing, while it does not cure colds and flu, it reduces their severity and the time they last by an average of about 40 percent. It does this by stimulating the immune system. In addition, zinc is part of super oxide dismutase, an effective antioxidant. In this capacity, and in conjunction with 200 or more different enzymes, zinc helps in almost every bodily function. For example, it increases sperm count, reverses male infertility, and helps prevent prostate problems.

Many people do not get as much zinc as the need. First of all, our bodies absorb only about 10 percent of their zinc intake. Second, we are unlikely to eat enough of zinc-containing foods to provide the full amount we need. While chicken, turkey, most forms of beans, ground beef, beef liver, pecans and cashews, Swiss cheese and yogurt contain zinc, the quantities are not large enough to supply us with the full amount we need.

You can take zinc in the form of zinc gluconate, zinc picolinate, zinc citrate, or zinc monomethionate. There is no evidence to suggest that any of these is better than the others.

We recommend 15 milligrams of whichever you choose daily.

OTHER SUPPLEMENTS

Of course, there are many other vitamins and minerals that can be helpful—and in some cases essential—to your health and the health of your skin. However, we believe the above regimen is optimal, and we do not recommend additional supplementation. We have two reasons for limiting your daily intake of supplements to those mentioned (and summarized in the list below):

1. The list of supplements we recommend already seems lengthy—although you will find that you can buy combination products that contain most of the supplements we recommend. If you start with an all-in-one product, you can then add those items that it either doesn't contain at all or contains in insufficient quantities.

2. There are several other vitamins and supplements that we have not included in our list, not because they are less important but because they are in abundant supply in food (even if you do not stick to a particularly healthy diet). Thus, the chance of your facing a nutritional deficit in anything other than the products mentioned above is negligible.

In this context it is worth emphasizing that there is no point in taking more of a particular vitamin or mineral than your body requires. With rare exceptions, the excess is simply eliminated, and you will have achieved nothing by taking more than you need (except a small depletion in your pocketbook). However, there are a few supplements that, taken to excess, may have limited negative side effects. So always be careful not to exceed our recommended dosages—and, before you take anything, always check with your physician.

SUMMARY

As noted, we recommend taking a branded multivitamin and then adding the extra items you may need to insure that every day you are taking the following vitamins and minerals:

Recommended Daily Supplement Intake	
Vitamin C	1,000–5,000 mg (the more the older you are)
Alpha lipoic acid	100 mg (if you are over 40)
Vitamin B complex	100 mg
Folic acid	Follow your doctor's advice. Extra for pregnant women
Vitamin E (tocotrienol/HPE)	200–800 IU (take more the older you are)
L-carnitine	1,000 mg
Calcium	1,000 mg
Magnesium	200 mg
Selenium	200 mcg
Chromium	200 mcg
Zinc	15 mg

We are confident that, after you have followed the routine of taking the supplements daily for a period of 2 to 3 months, you will start to experience renewed energy, and you may see an improvement in your general physical appearance and in the appearance of your skin in particular. If you can combine this new health regimen with a limited amount of extra exercise, you will find that the exercise is far more effective than you have experienced in the past. You may also find yourself losing weight. People may comment that you look less tired. And you can be reasonably sure that, in combination with the skin care program we discussed in chapter 6, you will never again suffer from acne.

But all these advantages, not inconsiderable in themselves, pale before the fact that, by following this regimen, you can be confident of living a longer, healthier, more energetic, and more attractive life.

8

ACNE IN MEN

MEN TEND TO SUFFER MORE FROM ACNE than do women.

There are several reasons for this, both physical and psychological. Fortunately, however, once the acne is cured, most of the problems dissipate.

The three most common causes of male distress from acne are:

1. The psychological impact of an acne-blemished face

2. The problem of ingrown hairs

3. Difficulty with shaving

There is a fourth problem that applies primarily to teenage boys that we shall deal with in a moment. First, however, let us deal with each of the three universal—and largely resolvable—issues in turn.

THE PSYCHOLOGY OF DATING

Both men and women, and especially young men and women, are typically deeply anxious about their relationships with the opposite sex. In particular, young people of both genders are shy and nervous, often to an extreme degree, about asking a person for a date.

Even making an initial attempt to *meet* someone can be a challenge.

However, even in today's attitudes of equality, the fact remains that, for the most part, the male makes—and is expected to make—the initial approach. That isn't to say that women can't or don't or shouldn't; it's just the condition of our cultural mores that men usually take the first step. (Thankfully, in today's world of Internet dating, this situation appears to be changing so that women are starting to be on a more equal footing—but they're not there yet.)

It is also true, as noted earlier, that acne sufferers typically assess the severity of their symptoms much more harshly than do objective observers.

When these two considerations merge, the result is that men, especially young men, viewing their acne as "awful" or "disgusting," are inhibited from approaching girls for a date. Even though a girl, viewing the problem as much less aversive than the man, might well accept a date, if she is never asked, she is not likely to initiate the contact. Consequently, and unnecessarily, the young man—and therefore the young woman—remains dateless.

On the other hand, boys will continue to ask girls out in spite of the girls' equally "awful" acne, for a variety of reasons. For one thing, as objective observers, they don't find the acne nearly as "disgusting" as the girls assume. For another, the girls can hide much of the problem with makeup. And, probably most important of all, the male libido is such that it is hardly going to be put off by anything as superficial, temporary, and limited as acne!

None of this is to imply that untreated acne is not a major problem for both sexes. It is. However, as you will understand by now, there is no need for the problem to remain untreated. And clearly, once the acne is cured, the issue becomes moot.

Of course, if the acne has already wreaked its havoc and major scarring remains, then at least part of the psychological harm remains with it. We will deal next with the temporary methods men can use to minimize the unsightliness—and hence the psychological impact—of scarring. (In chapter 12, we will discuss how scarring can be permanently reduced or eliminated through various surgical techniques.)

CAMOUFLAGING THE ACNE

For women, makeup can be an effective and, correctly used, harmless way of covering acne during the weeks it may take for the Acne Cure program to become fully effective. In addition, makeup can hide all but the most egregious scars from earlier acne.

However, men can hardly avail themselves of this solution. Fortunately, however, they enjoy some solutions unique to themselves.

Over the past few years, the "semi-shaved" look, pioneered by a number of Hollywood leading men, has become trendy among today's fashionable men. Even in the most conservative business circles, men with several days' stubble are not an uncommon sight. We have seen senior bankers, successful lawyers, and even an occasional politician sport this look.

According to a confidential study conducted by a major toiletries company, men who sport the unshaved look are considered by their peers to be "masculine or manly," "bold," "daring," "fashionable," "up-to-date," and "with it." Since these are qualities desirable in most professions, we suggest that the unshaved look, in addition to covering up acne scars, may also enhance the wearer's total appeal and reputation.

The semi-shaved look, possibly combined with a beard or mustache, brings three signal benefits with it. The first is that it is a fine cover for even unsightly blemishes or scars. Second, and less obvious, it has the advantage of letting men judiciously apply a limited amount of a skin-colored concealer over their blemishes or scars. Blended into the skin where red spots or scars would otherwise show, and then camouflaged by the "unshaved" hair, both the concealer and the acne become invisible.

The third and greatest bonus from this look is that men don't need to shave as frequently or as closely. That will undoubtedly reduce the problem in that it allows the man to avoid aggravating the pimples by inadvertently cutting into them, and to reduce the incidence of ingrown hairs.

INGROWN HAIRS

We stated a moment ago that *most* of men's acne problems disappear once the acne is cured. However, one problem remains: Ingrown hairs on the face and, to a more limited extent, in the pubic area, on the back, on the neck, and occasionally even on arms and legs can be a real problem. Facial ingrown hairs are a special difficulty for teenage boys. However, many men, particularly those with tightly curled or curly hair, continue to suffer from this problem throughout their lifetime.

Hairs grow from a spot in the subcutaneous layer just below the dermis where there is a small "bulb" surrounded by a group of capillaries whose blood nourishes the hair. The hair shaft grows from this bulb through the follicular canal and emerges at its exit (a pore). The hair is kept lubricated and hence glossy and healthy-looking by the sebum generated by the sebaceous gland attached to the hair near the bottom of the follicular canal.

Each hair grows for 2 to 5 years, then breaks off and falls out. The hair "bulb" then goes into a resting period of about 3 months; thereafter, a new hair follicle starts to grow.

The hairs themselves consist of several layers of keratin—essentially the same material as the stratum corneum—that interlock a bit like roof tiles. Even though keratin is a very durable and hard material, once it has emerged through the stratum corneum a hair is unlikely to reenter the skin even if it curls back on itself, because the stratum corneum protecting the skin's surface is just as hard. That is why you rarely find ingrown hairs on the skull, even on men with the curliest hair. Under certain conditions, however, instead of growing through the follicular canal and out of a pore, the hair may turn inward and penetrate the skin below the protective stratum corneum layer. Usually this happens in one of three circumstances:

1. If the emerging hair is very curly, it may turn spontaneously before ever reaching the skin's surface. Some hairs even grow in circles or whorls so that they cause circular ingrowths that can be quite painful.

2. If a comedonal acne wad blocks the hair from emerging, the hair may take the path of least resistance and turn inward.

3. If the hair has emerged properly, but a very sharp, well-constructed razor first pushes the skin out of the way and then cuts the hair as far down as it can reach, the hair may actually be cut below the stratum corneum. In this case, particularly if the end of the hair has been sliced into a sharp edge, the hair may catch on the bottom of the stratum corneum and thus be forced to change direction, going inward instead of outward.

Once a hair is growing inward, down through the epidermis and even into the dermis, the body reacts by rushing blood in—that is, by "inflaming" the area in an attempt to "cure" the invasion. However, extra white corpuscles, while effective in fighting off bacterial invasions, can obviously do nothing to fight off an ingrown hair. Thus, eventually, a different protective mechanism takes over: The body surrounds the foreign matter (in this case the ingrown hair) with a pus-like liquid designed to push or float the foreign object out.

While we tend to think of pus as a noxious material, it is actually the body's positive response to a problem. It consists of white blood cells, fibrin, various proteins, a number of other infection fighters, oil, and water, and its task is to flush out the foreign matter that is irritating the area. So important to our skin's health (indeed, to our general health) is this function that, as far back as ancient Greece, this material we so dislike was known as "laudable pus."

The result of all this is that the area where the problem resides becomes bumpy and develops a series of sores, each of which can last days or even weeks. The effect is similar to that of acne, but of course it is not the same thing. In this respect, however, even professionals can be fooled because the rash that results from ingrown hairs is indeed related to acne in three ways.

1. Ingrown hairs are particularly common in men whose beards or other hair is just beginning to grow. With a lot of new hairs emerging, a percentage may well reenter the skin as described. But this is also a time when these young men are experiencing huge hormonal shifts and considerable stress. (There is no stress like teenage angst!) Thus, acne breakouts are at their height.

Often the two conditions coincide, and the whole problem is described as acne.

2. The second area of confusion arises from the fact that the comedonal plugs that are the main cause of acne lesions may also interfere with or even block the emergence of hair follicles, thus encouraging them to change direction and reenter the skin. Now you have a

double problem in roughly the same location. On the one hand, the comedone blocking the pore may give rise to a sebum balloon below the surface and the resultant acne, while at the same time, the body may be fighting the ingrown hair with a pustule. The result may be an aggravated sore that sufferers (and sometimes their physicians) describe merely as acne. This is the main reason that ingrown hairs are commonly said to *cause* acne. They don't; but they may share a joint causative comedone, and they are certainly likely to aggravate each other and make the combined condition very unpleasant.

3. Finally, the act of shaving will indiscriminately cut into both the bumps that result from acne and those generated by the ingrown hairs. Typically, sufferers will then equate the two conditions as if they were the same thing, although, in fact, this too is a misconception.

HOW TO "CURE" INGROWN HAIRS

For men who suffer from ingrown hairs and either like to be clean shaven or are obligated to be so by their jobs, shaving becomes a daily aggravation.

We cannot promise that our solution to the problem of ingrown hairs is as complete as the Acne Cure program is for acne. However, the good news is, we can promise that the situation can be so controlled as to remain at worst a nuisance, in most cases, a very minor nuisance. Just follow this simple three-step program.

Step 1: Eliminate Your Acne

The first step is the obvious one: use the Acne Cure program to eliminate all the acne from the area where ingrown hairs may be causing harm. That step alone will dramatically reduce the whole problem, for it will not only remove all those bumps, pimples, blackheads, and whiteheads that are caused by the acne, but it will also remove closed comedones that are at least a partial cause of the ingrown hair. In many cases, the problem will be entirely solved; in all cases, it will be greatly reduced. (No doubt, if the condition disappears, men will say that the Acne Cure program also cured the acne caused by their ingrown hairs. They will be technically incorrect, but "where ignorance is bliss, 'tis folly to be wise"!)

While the acne cure is underway but you still suffer from some remaining blemishes, shave as little as possible. When you must shave, press only very lightly, and try to avoid shaving over any open wounds or scabs. You can do this by placing your finger over the spot and shaving all around it. In addition to not cutting the sore area or damaging a scab, this also allows a small amount of beard to grow over the blemish, thus somewhat camouflaging it. Then, once the blemish is healed, shave over it very gently, hardly pressing at all. Don't worry if there are a few longer hairs left in the area . . . you can get to them tomorrow.

Step 2: Take Care of Your Skin

Once your acne is eliminated, make sure you keep your skin healthy. This will both help stop your acne from reappearing, and make shaving easier. You can optimize your skin's health easily enough by following the recommendations we made in chapter 6.

Above all, keep your skin well-moisturized with an oil-free moisturizer so that the stratum corneum remains soft enough for the hair follicle to push through it. Don't worry; whatever you do, the stratum corneum will never become so soft that the hair can reenter. Since using a moisturizer (with a high SPF factor) is desirable for everyone, this represents no additional effort on your part.

Step 3: Shave Correctly

The most important step in dealing with any remaining ingrown hairs is *don't shave so close.*

You can achieve this effect in two ways. One is to use an electric shaver, but don't press too hard on your skin. No electric shaver ever shaved as close as a wet razor, for the simple reason that there is a screen between the cutting edge of the electric shaver and the skin, and there is none with a wet razor.

The other approach is to use a wet razor with a single blade edge. Many excellent shaving products have several blade edges in one "blade." For example, Mach-3 by Gillette has three blades set one behind the other. The effect is to give you an exceedingly close shave: First the protective bar in front of the three-edged "blade" pushes the skin away from the hair, then each blade successively pushes the skin further down, letting its edge cut a little closer. After three such attacks, nearly every hair has been cut to below the skin line and, if you are prone to the problem, is ready to double back on itself and grow inward. Single-edge blades will give you a shave that is quite close enough.

If you follow these three recommendations, you are unlikely to have a serious problem with ingrown hairs. However, if you care to, you can make the whole shaving experience much pleasanter than it is for most men (and eliminate almost all remaining ingrown hair problems) by shaving correctly.

HOW TO WET SHAVE CORRECTLY

On average, men shave over 15,000 times in a lifetime, using 3,500 hours (or about 150 days) in the process. If we wet shave, many of us, even if we do not suffer from ingrown hairs, frequently do suffer the inconvenience and discomfort of nicks and cuts, razor burn, and shaving-induced rashes. With rare exceptions, all these aggravations are the result of incorrect shaving techniques. The fact is, most men shave on automatic pilot, never thinking about what they do and therefore repeating endlessly any bad shaving habits they learned when they first started to shave or picked up along the way.

The correct way of wet shaving is, therefore, worth learning and implementing. After all, it doesn't take much longer (if at all) to do the job right, and it's much more comfortable.

Here, then, are the steps we recommend.

Step 1: Wet the Beard

This is very important for it softens the beard and makes cutting it easier. An easier cut means that the blade is less likely to catch on the hair and so pull part of the skin around it onto its sharp surface causing a nick (or a series of tiny nicks that add up to razor burn).

You can best wet the beard by using comfortably hot water. Naturally, a shower is the best way to do this, but if that isn't practical, splash your face thoroughly with hot water over the sink. Then apply some pre shave oil. Finally, cover your face with shaving cream, rubbing it in (rather than simply laying it onto the skin's surface).

Step 2: Use the Correct Razor

As noted above, if you are prone to ingrown hairs, use a razor that carries blades with a single cutting edge. If ingrown hairs are not a problem, you can use double- or triple-edged blades. In all cases, however, make sure that the blades are sharp. Dull blades will pull at your hairs and skin and thus increase the chance of nicks and cuts.

Step 3: Shave with the Grain

You can easily feel in the direction in which your facial hair grows, i.e. its grain, by running your hand over your beard. For most men, the grain is primarily downwards, especially in the mustache area, but may run in a different direction on the cheeks and in the neck area.

Once you have established in which direction your hair grows, shave with the grain. If you have been doing the opposite, you will find that shaving with the grain is so smooth it may feel as if you are not shaving at all. You are. What you are no longer doing is pulling at your beard and thus pulling the surface of your skin upward where, like as not, its surface will be sliced off. The result of shaving with the grain is that your shave will be just a tad less close—which, as we have said, is all to the good. However, it will be quite close enough for you to look clean-shaven—and your skin will be nick and rash free.

Step 4: Follow the Skin's Natural Contours

Your razor is constructed so that the bar in front of the blade flattens the skin allowing the blade to cut the hair to the right length. If you pull your skin to flatten it, the bar on the razor will stretch it further and you will increase the chances of damaging the skin's surface or cutting the hair too short. Thus, it is better to let the razor glide easily over the contours of your face. You need only use one hand to shave; the one not holding the razor should be unemployed!

Step 5: Clean Your Razor

As you are shaving, the cut fragments of your beard, mixed with the shaving cream, gather on the head of your razor. If you do not rinse them off between strokes, some are likely to end up between your skin and the edge of the razor's blade. This means that, instead of a flat blade edge cutting the hairs uniformly, some parts of the blade edge will be closer to the skin than others. The result will be an uneven shave and the need to shave some areas several times, both increasing the likelihood of irritation and the chance of cutting some hairs too closely, thus increasing the likelihood of ingrown hairs.

Step 6: Apply Aftershave

Finally, apply an aftershave moisturizing cream (not an alcohol aftershave which will dry out your skin). If you don't like the fragrances of many men's aftershave products, use a standard fragrance-free moisturizer with a sun block.

HOW TO DRY SHAVE CORRECTLY

When you dry shave, you have less flexibility—and, for most men, fewer potential problems with nicks, cuts, razor burn, and general discomfort—than when you wet shave. However, three simple principles still apply (and for the same reasons as with wet shaving), namely:

1. Soften your beard before you shave by using a pre shave product to make sure the shaver "slides" over your hairs as it is cutting them.

2. Make sure your shaver is thoroughly clean before you shave.

3. Use a moisturizer after you shave.

CONCLUSION

Acne in men can be cured just as easily and completely as in women. However, ingrown hairs are a problem that applies almost exclusively to men. It can often be cured, always minimized, but not always entirely eliminated.

Scarring in men and women can be largely corrected (as we shall discuss later), and in women any remaining visible scars can be almost entirely camouflaged with makeup. Men can achieve a similar effect with the unshaved look and with a limited amount of concealing makeup.

However, for men who want to be clean-shaven and whose previous severe acne has left unsightly scars, there are two solutions. One, which we shall discuss later, is to remove or minimize the scars by dermabrasion or even more invasive, surgical techniques.

The other is to decide to live with some visible remnant of the earlier condition. Perhaps, in making this decision, men can take heart from the fact that, like it or not, men's lives tend to be less influenced by their physical beauty than are women's. Not just, but true. Walt Whitman said of President Lincoln that his face was "so awful ugly it becomes beautiful, with its strange mouth, its deep-cut, crisscross lines, and its doughnut complexion." No man today has to look that bad; but still, in spite of his appearance, Lincoln managed to get by!

9

SPECIAL CONSIDERATIONS FOR CURING ACNE IN BLACK, HISPANIC, AND ASIAN SKIN

IN THE FIRST SENTENCE OF HIS BOOK *ACNE IN BLACK WOMEN*, Neil Persadsingh, M.D., wrote, "Acne is a chronic disorder of the skin, which means that it will be with you for many years."[1]

Dr. Persadsingh, we beg to differ! Using the Acne Cure program, your Black patients will find that their acne will be with them for no longer than the next 6 weeks! The fact is that, just as in White skin, in almost every case . . .

Acne in Black skin can be cured in 6 weeks or less.

Even when the Acne Cure program doesn't work completely—a circumstance that is almost as rare in Black skin as the 5 percent of the time it occurs in White skin—it will dramatically reduce the severity of the remaining acne. And we'll tell you in chapter 11 how to get rid of any acne remnant.

THE CAUSES OF ACNE IN BLACK SKIN

The cause and development of acne in Black skin is exactly the same as in White skin. The pores become occluded at the surface or within the follicular tube by a mixture of dry skin cells and sebum. The sebaceous glands, attached to the hair follicles near their base, continue to produce sebum. Since it can't escape, the sebum balloons up inside the follicular canal. Eventually, the balloon either pushes out the blockage at the surface and the mess erupts onto the skin, or the balloon ruptures inward and causes a nasty, relatively long-lasting acne lesion. Finally, in trying to fight the infection, the body rushes blood to the area—and the resulting inflammation swells the skin's surface, thus closing other pores and spreading the disease.

However, while the basic development of the disease is the same in Black skin as in White, there are four important differences in Black skin that tend to make acne problems more severe.

Before we discuss these differences, however, we must issue a caveat. "Black" is a description that covers all "people of color," and that color may range from truly dark to barely darker than, say, tanned White skin. Thus, any statements we make about "Black" skin must be hedged to say that they apply in general only and not to the skin of every "Black" person.

Generally, the darker the skin, the more the special characteristics applicable to Black skin are likely to pertain. But there are many exceptions.

Acne development is influenced by genetic inheritance. And there is evidence that acne originated in North Africa among dark-skinned Arabs, or Moors (as they were usually called). Tribes of these people invaded Portugal and Spain and moved into Southwestern France where they stayed for several centuries before being finally driven out. As a result, broadly speaking, there are two types of southern European skin: that which is swarthy as a result of some distant Moorish heritage, and that which is much the same color and appearance but stems from the tribes that emanated from Greece and southern Italy. Both skin types are on the dark side, but the former is acne-prone, while the latter tends to be relatively acne-resistant.

Moreover, even within the category of "Black" African and Indian skin, considerable differences apply among individuals, with the characteristics we describe as typical of Black skin tending to be more pronounced in African "Blacks" than in Indian "Blacks."

Fortunately, this confusion of colors is not really a problem since it is usually easy enough for each person to judge where their particular skin condition lies, and then to apply the Acne Cure program appropriately.

As stated, Black skin differs from White skin in four respects:

1. Nearly always there are more sebaceous glands in Black skin, and they tend to be larger and to produce more sebum. Naturally, therefore, the whole process of acne development tends to be more frequent, faster, and more severe.

2. Black skin's stratum corneum, while generally thinner than that of White skin, is denser. That is to say, it contains more cells in its thickness. That means that there are more dead cells sloughing off— and more opportunity for them to combine with the excess sebum to cause blockages.

3. While Black skin has no more melanocytes—melanin-producing cells—than White skin, the melanocytes it has are larger and more active. The advantage of the extra melanin is that it blocks much of the UVB light and thus makes it less likely that a dark-skinned person will suffer from sunburn. However, it does not filter out UVA light (which can penetrate glass, 3 feet of water, and even some summer clothing) and therefore does not prevent eventual skin wrinkling. Moreover, this extra melanin production unfortunately carries with it a serious disadvantage: Even relatively mild excitation from inflammation causes dark skin to produce extra melanin, which causes fairly prominent dark spots on the skin (called post-inflammatory hyperpigmentation, or PIHP for short).

4. Finally, the inflammatory reaction in Black skin tends to be stronger, so the spread of acne is generally more rapid and the condition itself more virulent. Dr. Persadsingh warns that in Black skin even "a mild case of acne can trigger an extreme inflammatory reaction."[2] The reason that Black skin reacts like this is that, associated with the skin's high melanin content, inflammation triggers the production of a number of chemicals that are able to attack and degrade the skin's elastin. This leads to visible scarring (which occurs more often in Black skin than in White); PIHP and consequent dark spots; occasionally the opposite reaction (white spots called vitiligo); and, most unsightly of all, keloids, which, as mentioned, are raised dark spots that sometimes look almost like scabs.

The four conditions described above are notably different in Black and White skin. Hispanic skin lies somewhere in between. In addition, there are two conditions that are not different but occur more frequently in Black skin. One applies to Black men—namely that because Black hair tends to be curly and relatively thick, ingrown hairs (discussed in chapter 8) are much more common. In fact, according to some estimates, as many as 60 percent of all Black men suffer from ingrown hairs at least once in their lives, whereas among fairskinned men the incidence of acne is thought to be under 25 percent.

The other problem with Black skin is that scarring from acne is both more likely to occur and tougher to remove surgically. In a later chapter, we will discuss dermabrasion, laser peeling, and surgical techniques to remove post-acne scarring. Here, it is sufficient to say that all these techniques have to be handled with even greater care on Black than on White skin because, as a result of its high melanin content, Black skin scars more visibly, develops light or dark spots more easily, and reacts negatively to a wider range of topical treatments than does White skin.

DEMOGRAPHIC CONSIDERATIONS

In addition to the physiological differences between Black, Hispanic (or southern European), and White skin, there are several demographic differences that surprisingly have a significant impact on acne.

The first is that the Black population in the United States—and, to a lesser extent, the Hispanic populations (except for the Puerto Ricans in the New York area)—tend to be concentrated in areas where the climate is hotter and more humid. As you know, in these warmer climes, one tends to perspire more than in cooler areas. The act of sweating actually aggravates or increases the likelihood of acne as the excess moisture swells the skin around the pores, which blocks them, causing more acne. In other words, while Black skin is more prone to acne anyhow, it is also true that demographically Blacks often reside in "acne-genic" locations—that is, the areas of the country with high temperatures and humidity. This compounds their acne problem.

The second sociological factor is that Black men and Black women often use oil-containing hair products. These products are usually used to give added sheen and to help manageability. Since any oily product applied to the hair is likely to spread to adjacent areas, especially the forehead, neck, and upper shoulders (already acne-prone areas), these hair preparations often aggravate acne.

Black women (and very occasionally Black men) often straighten their hair, a procedure that generally involves the use of harsh chemicals. Also, certain curling techniques involve the use of chemicals and heat. We have no proof, but we suspect that some of these chemicals may slightly damage and dry the skin near the scalp, making it more prone to acne invasions.

Finally, more Blacks and Hispanics in the United States smoke than do Whites. And, as we discussed earlier, there is no doubt that smoking, in addition to all its other negatives, aggravates acne.

THE ACNE CURE FOR BLACK SKIN

The Acne Cure program works almost as well on Black skin as on White. (If the results are marginally poorer—for example, an estimated success rate of 90 percent rather than, as for Whites, 95 percent—it is because the acne problems in Black skin tend to be more severe than in White. As discussed above, Black skin may be more impacted both by smoking and by climatic conditions conducive to acne formation.)

To apply the Acne Cure program to Black skin, however, requires more care. Here are the specifics of the program for Black skin.

Step 1: Cleaning Away Excess Dead Cells

Remember that, on the one hand, the stratum corneum of Black skin tends to be thinner, while on the other, it tends to be denser. In addition, since the sebaceous glands in Black skin tend to produce more sebum, it is usually kept oilier.

The result is that, if you examine Black skin closely—especially darker African-American skin—you will see that it has a lovely reflective glow to it. Black skin, looked at closely (and stated without political overtones), is truly beautiful.

Specifically, Step 1 for the Acne Cure program breaks into two parts:

1. Cleanse your face thoroughly with a mild, oil-free cleanser. (Plain water will do if your face is not particularly dirty.)

2. Complete the cleansing with a 2% salicylic acid wash. Be especially careful not to use a stronger solution.

Step 2: Removing the Clog

The second step of the Acne Cure program is exactly the same for Black as for White skin: Apply glycolic acid, using exactly the same method as described earlier, in chapter 4.

While the treatment is the same as for White skin, Black skin enjoys a side benefit from glycolic acid. If your skin has suffered from post-acne discoloration, glycolic acid will probably improve the condition by blending the discoloration. Nothing short of surgery will make the scars go away. But with glycolic acid, they may retreat. In any case, the glycolic acid will be the effective second step in making sure that no new scars form.

We should add one minor caveat to the use of glycolic acid on Black skin. There is a possibility that, in stronger concentrations than we recommend, glycolic acid can bleach Black hair to a grayish tint. We doubt that this would occur at our proposed concentration, but we suggest nevertheless that you keep the product away from your hair.

Step 3: Stopping the Disease Dead in Its Tracks

The third step in curing acne in Black skin is similar to, but not quite the same as, that for White skin. That is because BP, the main reagent used for Step 3, may occasionally, leave brown spots on dark skin. Thus, before you start, make certain that the BP product you have purchased is at a concentration that *definitely* does not exceed 5.0%. Indeed, if you can find a product with a lower concentration, down to as little as 2.5%, that would be preferable. At this level, the product remains fully efficacious but carries little risk of causing discoloration. The (very limited) remaining risk will be further reduced if, before you apply the BP, you make sure that your whole face is very wet from the ice cubes.

Apply only a very thin layer of the benzoyl peroxide product. In even minimal quantities, BP will be effective in eliminating *P. acnes*, but the less you apply, the smaller will be the chance of discoloration. Then, gently but insistently, rub the product in all over your face, including those areas where you don't have any acne. The reason for wetting the whole face and then applying BP over all its surface is that, if you cover only part of it, you will likely "spill over" in some places and risk discoloration there. In any case, a massage of your whole face feels good even if you have to administer it to yourself. (If you're really lucky, maybe you can get someone else to do the massaging for you. That is heaven!)

At the completion of the massage, apply the cold pack in the normal way.

Step 4: Protecting Your Skin

Just because your skin is dark, and therefore far less likely to suffer from sunburn, does not mean that you should not use a sunblock. Black people often do not start getting significant numbers of visible facial wrinkles until they are in their forties, but, if they have not protected themselves against UVA light, they do get wrinkles. Obviously, this protection is more necessary for lighter skin, but it is desirable in everyone. Although of relatively less benefit in very dark skin, for people with other Black skin tones, protecting against ultraviolet light will stop wrinkling, maintain or recreate your skin's vital glow, reduce the chances that acne will reappear, and, if it does recur, make certain that it can be rapidly eliminated.

As for the rest of the maintenance program for Black skin, it is exactly the same as for White skin. Stick to it and in all likelihood you'll never view acne as a problem again.

DOUBLE-DOSING

Since Black skin is more acne prone, particularly if you live in a hotter or more humid climate, you may find that it does not respond to the Acne Cure program as quickly as you would like. If you do not see a significant improvement by the end of week 3 of applying the program, we suggest that you speed up the process. Apply the BP (including the cold treatment) twice a day, in the mornings (after you complete the other morning steps) as well as before you go to bed, leaving the rest of the program unaltered. Admittedly, that can be a nuisance since it means you have to spend 15 minutes or so extra every day. On the other hand, you will be surprised by how pleasant, relaxing, and calming a cool ice pack on your face can be for a few minutes before you go to work. And the payoff is worthwhile: Within a very short time, you will see your acne receding fast.

Some White patients have asked us whether doubling the treatment would speed up the results of the program on White skin. Sorry! It may still take up to 6 weeks because, at least for deep-rooted acne, the imbedded balloons of pus and sebum have to reach the surface, where they can be effectively attacked, before you are fully cured—and that may take time. Doubling up doesn't speed up the Acne Cure for Black skin—it just makes the program work better.

THE ACNE CURE FOR HISPANIC SKIN

According to James E. Fulton Jr., M.D., Ph.D., of the Fulton Skin Institute in Newport Beach, California, a leading expert on acne, the gene that caused cystic acne—the most severe kind—"came from a Mediterranean gene pool and was spread around the world by the early Spanish adventurers. When the Spanish came into the Philippines and intermarried, acne became an epidemic problem of those islands. When the Spanish Conquistadors went to Mexico . . . wherever they . . . penetrated . . . there remains the cystic acne problem."[3] Fortunately, however, by no means is all Hispanic skin equally prone to this problem. Where the Conquistadors had less impact on the local population—for instance, further inland, where there is a larger component of the Indian gene pool, or where they came from further north in Spain—inherited acne is both less widespread and less severe.

The treatment for acne in Hispanic skin is a matter of choice. In cases where the acne is not unusually severe and where the skin tone is lighter, you should follow exactly the protocol outlined in chapter 4.

In the rarer cases, where the skin is darker, the pores larger, and the acne more severe, you should treat it as per the modified treatment program described above for Black skin.

THE ACNE CURE FOR ASIAN SKIN

Asians as a rule have wonderful skin. It is more resistant to sun damage than White skin, but, compared with Black skin, it tends to have pores that are smaller and less likely to become clogged. Generally, therefore, Asian patients suffer less from acne in frequency and severity.

Indeed, these are the only disadvantages from which Asian skin (as compared with White skin) may suffer: It sometimes tends to become sallow; it may dry out and wrinkle more; and, in extreme cases of scarring from excessive abrasion or facial surgery, it may be somewhat more prone to discoloration.

Of course, the fact that acne in Asian skin is generally less of a problem than in most other types of skin does not mean that this generality applies to your particular case. What it does mean is that the Acne Cure program we have outlined in chapter 4 will work to eliminate acne in Asian skin more than 95 percent of the time. In the remaining situations, the methods described in chapter 11 will certainly resolve the problem.

CONCLUSION

For both physiological and demographic reasons, Blacks are more likely to develop acne than Whites, and it is likely to be more severe. Moreover, the aftereffects of severe acne are likely to be more visible on Black skin since, in addition to pitting and pocking (problems that appear equally in Black and White skin), Black skin may develop dark spots, light spots, keloids, or, in some particularly unfortunate cases, all three. In general, the frequency and severity of these problems roughly correlates with the darkness of the skin.

Conversely, although Asians may (rarely) suffer from discoloration problems, they generally suffer less from acne—and therefore less from acne scarring—than do people with other skin tones.

Given this information, it is clear that the Acne Cure program is even more important for dark-skinned acne sufferers than for those with lighter skin. Happily, it works almost as well on even the darkest skin as it does on porcelain-colored White skin. The only practical difference is that for Black skin the program has to be applied with a degree of delicacy that is hardly needed on other skin types. Once that is done, it works almost as effectively. At least 9 out of 10 cases of even the severest acne on even the darkest of skin will be gone within no more than 6 weeks from the start of the cure.

10

STRESS

HERE IS THE CONUNDRUM about stress and acne: On the one hand, there is no doubt that stress increases the likelihood of your suffering an acne outbreak. On the other hand, highly successful people—who typically work competitively, accept challenges, take risks, and in general place themselves in stressful situations—do not seem to suffer excessively from acne. As we look at World Series or Super Bowl athletes, political candidates in do-or-die debates, astronauts entering their space capsules, or young entrepreneurs negotiating their first big deal, we don't see a sea of zits. Those faces may be full of determined tension, but their skin is clear.

Stress is associated not only with acne but with a long line of grave diseases, including:

• Suppression of the reproductive system, causing impotence in men, a cessation of menstruation (amenorrhea) in women, and a reduction of the libido in both

• Inflammatory symptoms in the lungs contributing to asthma, bronchitis, and a variety of other respiratory diseases

• Suspension of tissue repair, contributing to osteoporosis

• Strain on the pancreas that may become a factor in adult-onset (Type II) diabetes

• Increase in chronic pain associated with a variety of diseases, including arthritis

• Inhibition of several immune system components that increase susceptibility to flu, cancer, and even AIDS.

It seems that some people facing exceedingly high levels of stress are somehow unaffected. Yet others, facing no more than such largely psychological factors as imagined threat, noise, or even crowding, may feel themselves harshly pressured—and may indeed break out in acne.

Stress and its management is a field replete with such contradictions and conundrums.

As you read stress management books, you will see that, for the most part, their authors recommend that to control your stress, you should teach yourself different habits—that is, you should change your lifestyle.

Even if it were true that you could stop competing and still win the competition, stop worrying about achievement but still achieve, stop being impatient but still get as much done, or stop rushing and still win the race, do you really want to change your personality (even if that were possible, which we seriously doubt) or fundamentally modify your lifestyle in order to relieve your acne? Seems a bit extreme, doesn't it?

If you find yourself in a situation where the stress you feel is making you unhappy, depressed, and sick *and* is aggravating your acne, then it's time to do something about it. That's "bad stress," and if you care to deal with it, you will solve many of your problems, including your risk of recurring acne attacks. We'll deal in a moment with how to deal with bad stress.

On the other hand, if you are feeling stressed because you are about to get married, you'll hardly want to give up that idea just because it's causing your face to break out. For one thing, you now know how to cure the acne regardless of how much stress you face. For another, this is good stress. After we deal with the bad version, we will provide you with some suggestions on how you can make your good stress even better.

The fact is, as is elegantly emphasized by Martha Davis, Ph.D., and her coauthors, in their perennially best-selling book *The Relaxation and Stress Reduction Workbook*, "Stresses are often positive. . . . The physical exertion of a good workout, the excitement of doing something challenging for the first time, or the pleasure of watching a beautiful sunset are all examples of positive stress."[1]

Moreover, there is considerable evidence that, up to a point, even bad stress can be helpful. Performance improves as stress mounts. We are able to muster the adrenaline for the final sprint of the marathon more easily if we hear our competitors pounding at our heels than if we are all alone way ahead of the pack. We are better able to concentrate on getting the paper written as its deadline approaches. And we can undertake feats of remarkable courage and endurance when necessity dictates.

But while increasing stress increases performance, once the stress becomes excessive, performance plummets. Like many other animals, at the first sign of danger we either cleverly scamper away or, intelligently assessing our chances, prepare to fight. But, like those animals, if the stress of the danger becomes too great, we either freeze into useless immobility or blindly flee in equally useless panic.

Of course, in our modern world, while all our animalistic impulses continue to apply, we rarely actually fight or flee, even when our stress reaches panic levels. For example, young executives ready to make a major presentation to a panel of their bosses, or novice actors about to go onstage on opening night, quite often either vomit or suffer an acute attack of diarrhea. Each of these reactions is an age-old remnant of our earlier existence, when our bodies prepared to fight or flee by emptying themselves of excess weight. But presenting the annual marketing plan or reciting the prologue to Hamlet, however stressful, would hardly be aided by temporary weight reduction.

WHY IS STRESS HARMFUL?

To understand how to deal with stress, we should first understand why it is harmful.

When one of our prehistoric ancestors faced a sudden challenge (be it the danger of being attacked by some larger and faster predator or the opportunity to slay a larger and faster prey), his body prepared for action in a number of ways.

As stated, the body eliminated unnecessary weight. But it also pumped out adrenaline, raised blood sugar levels, speeded up breathing, heart, and metabolism rates, increased muscle tension, and raised blood pressure. Once the needed elimination was complete, the body of a prehistoric man locked down his intestines so that he would not be disturbed by elimination needs while he was fighting or fleeing. His pupils dilated and his hearing acuity increased so that he could see and hear his enemy or prey more clearly. The more effectively his body responded, the more likely he was to avoid the danger or to catch his supper. Those whose responses were mild died earlier and reproduced less. The survivors were those who had the stronger responses to stress. And, of course, it is from that surviving gene pool that we are descended. No wonder stress affects us.

Prehistoric stress reactions were positive because all the preparations the body made were needed, indeed vital, for survival. Saving oneself from danger or hunting for one's sustenance inevitably involved vigorous physical effort. And that effort used up the excess adrenaline and blood sugar, tired out (and thus relaxed) tense muscles, expended the extra energy generated by accelerated metabolism, and burned off the extra oxygen the speeded-up breathing had provided. After a short time, the excess energy generated as a stress response that allowed our ancestors to survive had been used up. Their bodies rapidly returned to their normal equilibrium.

However, stress as we experience it today rarely requires a physical response. Thus, when the cerebral cortex (the conscious, thinking part of the brain) senses a stressful situation, it sends the age-old alarm to the hypothalamus (the "instinctive," reactive part of the brain). That, in turn, stimulates the sympathetic nervous system to make all the stress-related adjustments it has made since time immemorial.

Of course, once the stress ends, a relaxation response steps in. Not only does the body stop producing the stress-related stimulants; it gradually absorbs and dissipates any remaining unneeded ones. After all, even ancient man might have sensed danger and prepared for it only to discover it was a false alarm. Thus, occasional overstimulation of the fight-or-flight reaction is not harmful.

However, today's world is different in two respects: One is that, although we endure repeated stress alarms, we rarely if ever have to respond physically; the other is that much of our stress may continue for long periods, often semipermanently. Unlike the athlete whose stress response starts at the beginning and ends at the conclusion of the game, many of us, facing the daily stress of work or money shortage or family problems, never turn those stresses off. For both these reasons, for many people, the stress reaction is almost continual. We even suffer from nightmares or wake up in the middle of the night, filled with anxiety about how to pay tomorrow's bills.

As a result, the adrenaline and other energy-producing chemicals secreted by the adrenal glands have a negative effect. Rather than shutting down various bodily operating systems—and increasing blood sugar, adrenaline, etc.—for just long enough for us to deal physically with whatever is causing the stress, they continue to do so over long periods. Eventually, this continuing overstimulation without release (somewhat akin to racing your engine with your foot firmly on the brake) may do permanent damage. Overexerting the pancreas gland—necessary to deal with the unutilized sugar in the blood—may lead to hypoglycemia and eventually diabetes; unrelenting extra blood pressure may lead to hypertension and heart disease; and the continuous strain of adrenaline-like stimulants may undermine the immune system.

There is no doubt that stress has a whole raft of negative impacts on the body. In fact, it has been found to be a significant factor not only in all the diseases mentioned previously but also in the development of depression. And, amid all of these problems, as if they were not serious enough, stress also aggravates acne.

SOLVING STRESS

As we have already pointed out, eliminating stress from our daily lives is impractical for most of us, and undesirable for many of us. We thrive on stress. We need it to motivate ourselves.

No, we do not wish to banish stress if it contributes to the success in our lives. Rather, the trick is to learn to view stress differently—as a positive feeling, not a negative one. This is an act of modern will, just as it is by an act of modern will that, when facing a crisis, we choose to solve it in ways that involve neither fleeing nor fighting.

You cannot avoid blinking if someone throws a pretend punch at your face, even though you know it's an experiment and that the person has no intention of touching you. But you can avoid ducking your head and throwing up your arms in self-defense or clenching your fists, ready to counterattack. The result is that the instinctive blink has almost no effect on your internal chemical makeup. Similarly, you can teach yourself to accept the permanent stressors in your life as positive and stimulating rather than negative and harmful.

In the phrase introduced by stress researcher Suzanne Kobasa, M.D., of the University of Chicago, you can become "stress hardy."

Training Your Body's Stress Reaction

Stress reduction techniques fall into two main categories:

1. Those that concentrate on reducing stress levels by teaching you how to change your behavior.

2. Those that teach you how to view your stress as positive and thus avoid its harmful side effects.

In the next few pages, we will deal with both approaches. However, we should emphasize that we consider the second approach to be generally the more useful. A new job, marriage and divorce, looming exams or presentations, performance anxiety—nearly always such stressors are either desirable or unavoidable. And most have their upsides (yes, even divorce, which, after all, can be viewed as the end of a problematic situation). Looking at each problem from a positive perspective should allow us to convert them from bad to good stress, and thus from a disease- and acne-producing condition to a health- and vitality-stimulating one.

UNDERSTANDING YOUR BODY'S STRESS

Since your body reacts instinctively to stress, you may not be sufficiently aware of the stress you are carrying around with you, or what generates it. As Dr. Davis put it, "Most people are more aware of the weather, the time of day, or their bank balance than they are of the tension in their own bodies or their personal stress response."[2] But of course if you are not aware of your stress, you will not be able to do much about it.

To find out what stresses you suffer from and what causes them, we suggest you keep a "tension diary" for a few weeks. This is a simple task: On a standard sheet of lined, $8\frac{1}{2}$-by-11-inch paper, make three columns. The left-hand column shows the hours of the day you are awake (including hours you cannot sleep at night). The easiest way to do this is to leave spaces for 24 hours, and then leave blank those hours that you are asleep.

In the middle column, write a brief description of the stressful event that took place during each hour (late for work; important client presentation; cocktail party—and I hate cocktail parties—and so on). If there was no stressful event during a certain hour, leave the line blank.

In the right-hand column, describe any negative *physical* or emotional symptoms you experienced during each hour (such as mild headache, backache, nausea, diarrhea, insomnia; anger, depression, sadness). Again, if you feel nothing significant during any given hour, leave the space blank.

Prepare a new sheet each day. After a while, you will see a pattern forming—actually, two patterns. One pattern will be of repeating stressful behaviors. Often you cannot (or do not wish to) make changes in these. The weekly briefing you make to the chairman may be nerve-racking in the extreme, but it is also moving your career forward rapidly. Occasionally, however, you may detect a situation you can change. "Late for train" every day may be resolved by getting up 10 minutes earlier.

The second, more useful pattern you will see is which of these apparently stressful events are regularly followed by negative reactions (and which are not). Perhaps that stressful chairman's briefing is rarely if ever followed by any negative symptoms, whereas paying bills usually engenders a headache.

Changing Behaviors

Although we do not generally endorse changing behaviors as being a practical way of alleviating stress, there are certainly instances where this is not only possible but realistic. If your tension diary shows that, indeed, "late for train" happens day after day and is palpably causing you negative stress-related symptoms, you may be able to reset your schedule to start the day a little earlier.

One friend of ours, facing this circumstance, just couldn't wake up and get himself going until a deadline was upon him. Self-delusion to the rescue: Instead of getting up "earlier," our friend set all the clocks in his house to be a few minutes fast. He figured that he'd thus be able to get up at the "same" time as always, but with a few more minutes to get ready. That worked for him, provided he wasn't sure just how fast his clocks actually were. If he knew exactly, the delusion would fail: He would mentally discount the extra time and still find himself late. To combat this, he set his clocks with his eyes closed, giving the minute hand on the face of each clock a minor twist forward, but never knowing by how much. He was rarely late again.

Nevertheless, symptoms of stress generally cannot be overcome by changing lifestyles. To do so would cause stress-related problems of omission that would probably be worse than those from the stress they were trying to resolve. Rather, in most cases, the better method of dealing with stress is to leave it intact but consider it from a different angle.

CHANGING YOUR PERSPECTIVE
ON STRESS

Stress is inevitable.

And so are its symptoms. For example, virtually every one of us lives with more tension in our muscles than we could possibly need for any physical exertion in which we are likely to participate. To prove this to yourself, try this simple exercise.

1. Lie down and get comfortable on a relatively flat surface—it's okay if your knees are bent or even if you are half lying on a recliner, just as long as your feet are level with or above your head. Relax in the normal way—that is, letting your body go limp.

2. Breathe in deeply. Then let the air out slowly and as completely as you can, concentrating on relaxing your chest, breathing through your diaphragm, and letting your stomach "collapse."

As you let that deep breath out, in all likelihood you will feel your shoulders—indeed the whole of your upper torso—relaxing even if you thought you were relaxed before you started. (Evidently, you had tensed those muscles more than you realized.) Try the exercise two or three more times, and you will find more and more tension ebbing away.

3. Try to relax each arm and leg in turn, taking a deep breath before each event. You'll see that, here too, you will find a considerable additional reduction in muscle tension each time you let out your breath—there, that's proof that you are under tension!

Of course, much of the continuing tension we all feel is desirable. For example, if you stayed in the advanced state of relaxation that you induced while you were doing this exercise, you surely wouldn't get much done. That's a good position to be in if you're on vacation at the beach (wearing plenty of sunblock, off course!), but it's hardly practical for your workaday life. Indeed, the purpose of the exercise was largely to show you just how much tension you carry permanently—most of which you actually need.

To learn to live with this tension—that is, to maintain its desirable attributes while eliminating its negative ones—we recommend the following simple steps.

Step 1: Taking a Tension Inventory

We believe it is important that you start by taking your tension inventory (with a tension diary, as described earlier) so that you know accurately with what tension-producing circumstances you are dealing.

Then eliminate any that are not needed or wanted in your regular life.

Step 2: The 10-Minute Relaxation

Set aside 10 minutes a day for relaxation. Don't try for much more than that unless you feel like it; you are a busy person, and taking more time than that away from your full day is just as likely to increase your tension as to reduce it. Of course, while you are still curing your acne, the 10 minutes you need for cooling your face and applying the BP can double as your relaxation time. (In the future, even though your acne is cured, you may enjoy the cooling effect enough to want to continue to use it during your daily relaxation period.)

During this time, learn to relax *efficiently*. There are specific techniques to do this; some authors have written books on the subject. Frankly, learning to relax—at least to the level you will find useful—

is not that hard. ("Working to relax" has always struck us as an oxymoron!) Here is what we recommend.

1. Find a comfortable chair in a peaceful location, or at least one where you are not likely to be interrupted. (You don't need silence; for example, most people can relax very nicely in an airplane, provided their neighbor doesn't insist on chatting.)

2. Turn on your favorite *soothing* music; this is no time for hip-hop, heavy metal, or, if classical music arouses you, Beethoven's fifth.

3. Spend a minute or so observing your own breathing rhythms.

STRESS BUSTERS

Given that stress is something that we must learn to deal with effectively, on a day-in-and-day-out basis—and especially at work—here are three anti-stress exercises that we have found helpful. You can do them at your desk, they don't interfere with your workday, and (the best part) more than likely they will give you an energy boost.

• **Neck stretches.** While sitting in your chair, tip your head from side to side, then forward, and then backward. Repeat a few times.

• **Forward stretches.** While sitting in your chair, stretch your body forward, letting your head and arms come forward. Hold for 30 seconds, and then straighten up. Repeat.

• **Shoulder rolls.** Raise your shoulders toward your ears. Drop your shoulders. Slowly rotate your shoulders forward, then backward.

Once you are aware of your breathing, slow it down and deepen it somewhat. Don't exaggerate this; just breathe a shade more slowly and deeply than you normally would—to simulate the rhythm of your breathing when you are asleep.

4. Next, concentrate on each part of your body in turn, starting with your toes and feet and working up to your face (where you will probably find permanent tension in your lips, cheeks, forehead, eyebrows, and lids). As you concentrate on each body part, first tense the muscles as hard as you can without moving from your supine position. Then take in a medium-deep breath. Finally, blow out your breath as completely as you can while concentrating on relaxing the tensed muscles in that body part as much as possible. Repeat this two or three times.

5. Now that you are considerably more relaxed than usual and your breathing is slower and deeper, visualize a soothing environment, perhaps a quiet garden you know or a sleepy Sunday morning in bed—any situation you associate with calm and wellbeing. The main purpose of this exercise is not to transport you to a different location but to stop you for a few minutes from thinking about your everyday problems and concerns. Alternatively, if you prefer, you can use the meditation technique of concentrating on a single word, object or color, or saying the word aloud, a mantra.

Obviously, you will fail to block out all other thoughts. However hard you try, they will insinuate themselves, including the inevitable thought that you are failing at this exercise. Never mind. As soon as you find yourself straying, just force your mind back to your simple image, word, or color. In so doing, you will be very effectively using your mind to block out the worries and ambitions upon which you (necessarily and desirably) concentrate during the rest of the day.

By the time you have finished this exercise, you will feel greatly refreshed. More important, by putting your troubles on hold for a few minutes, you will unconsciously have also put them into perspective. How bad could those problems be if you can wipe them from your mind so completely, even for a short time? (If you have truly grievous problems, this technique won't work. Some problems cannot be ignored even for a few minutes. Nothing will help but the alleviation of the problems. Therefore, it is solely to that end that you should expend all your time and energy.)

Step 3: Gaining Perspective

Once a week, compose a written list of the problems you expect to face during the coming week. There will be two aspects of this: One will be the specific tensions you have identified from your tension diary; the other will be more general problems—for example, the long-term illness of a loved one or your chronic shortage of money.

Then, considering each of these "life's problems," figure out with respect to each what would be the worst thing that could realistically happen. Your loved one could die. You could be bankrupted or perhaps find yourself homeless.

Once you understand your worst-case scenarios, compare them with the actual situation you face. Inevitably, you will realize—or reaffirm—either that your situation is not nearly as bad as it could be or that the problem is already so severe that it cannot get much worse. In either case, you will gain a sense of relief.

Thinking about your problems rationally—and thus either developing ways to solve them or coming to terms with their inevitability—rather than inchoately worrying about them is a well-established technique for reducing tension.

ENSURING GOOD SLEEP

Getting a good night's sleep can be a significant stress reducer for those who are overworked and tired a good deal of the time. In any case, while establishing effective sleeping patterns may not completely rid you of stress, it will take the edge off the feelings of stress you may have. Here are some "good sleep hygiene" tips from *Self-Help* magazine.[3]

- Go to bed when you are actually sleepy or tired—not when it's "time to go to bed."

- Once you are in bed, turn out the light with the clear intent of going to sleep. Don't read or watch television in bed. Make sure your body reacts automatically (like Pavlov's dog to the sound of a bell) to bed by associating it with sleeping. (The exception to this, of course, is that bed is also for giving each other a massage, cuddling, and making love. Those are all relaxants that will help you sleep.)

- Wind down during the evening hours before bedtime. So try to stay away from anxiety-provoking or mentally or physically stimulating activities for at least $1\frac{1}{2}$ hours before going to bed. Block anxious thoughts by doing something interesting enough to hold your attention, but not exciting. Crossword puzzles are a good example.

- Use the "relax efficiently" technique described above. A good time for this is just as you get into bed.

- Keep your room cool.

- Reserve exercise for the morning or afternoon.

- Don't nap during the day.

And one final piece of advice for you insomniacs for whom none of the above seems to help:

A friend of ours just couldn't stay asleep for more than 3 or 4 hours at a time. He would wake up in the middle of the night and lie there, tossing and turning, until dawn—only to fall into a deep slumber just minutes before the wake-up alarm shrilled. Of course, all day long he would feel exhausted, hardly able to complete the day's tasks.

Eventually, close to desperation, he visited a renowned sleep expert. "What can I do? I'm tired all the time. I can barely handle my job," our friend lamented.

The expert checked him thoroughly for both physical and mental problems but found nothing substantive wrong. In the end, he gave him a list of sleep hygiene tips much like the ones above.

"And if they don't work and I still can't sleep?"

"Get up and do your work," the expert replied.

"But then I'll feel tired in the morning."

The great expert glowered at him. "So?" he demanded.

We met our friend a few weeks later and asked how he was feeling.

"Exhausted," he told us with a happy grin. "But I'm all caught up on my work."

CONCLUSION

Anxiety disorder is becoming a more widely recognized mental disease. For example, *Time* magazine's cover story in its June 10, 2002, issue was on this condition. If you are among those unfortunate people who experience its symptoms, you need medical assistance. You should never try to treat yourself. Not only are you probably not an expert in the field, but even if you are, how can you use your brain to fix the shortcomings from which that same brain is suffering? It would be like an eye surgeon trying to stare into a mirror while operating on his own eyes.

However, if you experience only a normal level of anxiety and tension—in other words, if you are just like most of us—you can control the negative effects of that tension.

We are not suggesting that if you follow the simple steps outlined in this chapter, your life will become tension-free. We doubt that a tension-free life is feasible or even desirable. However, you will find that you can greatly reduce the level of the bad tension you feel by the simple means we have outlined. In doing so, you will improve the quality of your days, perhaps a great deal. At the same time, as a sort of bonus, you will greatly reduce your susceptibility to renewed acne attacks.

11

CURING
INTRACTABLE ACNE

IN THEIR BOOK *SKIN DEEP*, Carol Turkington, M.D., and Jeffrey Dover, M.D., identify no fewer than 14 different types of acne in addition to acne vulgaris, the main target for the Acne Cure program this book describes. To prove their academic credentials, they give them all Latin names![1]

However, many of these different types of acne turn out to be merely variations on vulgaris brought on by varying external conditions. Thus, they can all be easily resolved. In some cases the solution is even easier because this involves no more than eliminating the cause; in others (particularly when the cause cannot be easily eliminated), it means eradicating the acne by the protocol we have outlined. Sometimes, the most rapid cure involves both removing the cause and applying our cure.

Four of the types are rarer but also more intractable forms of acne. It is usually among these that are to be found the 5 percent of acnes that will be helped but not completely eliminated by the Acne Cure program. As we have mentioned, they generally appear in conjunction with vulgaris.

In the balance of this chapter, we will first describe those acnes that, like acne vulgaris, can be cured in virtually all cases within a 6-week time frame by the application of our program and then discuss those acnes whose resolution may require additional medication.

For purposes of simplification, we have condensed the list prepared by Turkington and Dover into two sets: the following nine, which are little more than variations on acne vulgaris and can therefore be almost entirely eliminated by the Acne Cure program, and the subsequent four, which may call for sterner medical treatment.

VARIATIONS ON ACNE VULGARIS

Acne vulgaris has nine variations, which we will describe here.

Acne Cosmetic

As we shall discuss elsewhere, cosmetics rarely if ever cause acne. However, cosmetics that are particularly greasy or oily may be a contributing factor. Try to avoid them.

If you are not sure whether or not the makeup you are using is oily (labels and cosmeticians' advice sometimes being subject to what Winston Churchill once called "terminological inexactitude"), place a small drop of your makeup onto a standard piece of typing paper, work it around until it is about the size of a dime, and leave it overnight. By the next morning, you will see a ring of grease around the makeup. If its width is more than a quarter of the diameter of the makeup "blob," the makeup contains more oil than you probably need.

In their book, Turkington and Dover also identified pitch acne (caused by coal tar shampoos) and pomade acne (caused by oily hair pomade, which we mentioned previously as a problem faced primarily by Black men). Changing to a different product (an antidandruff shampoo, such as Head and Shoulders, that is not based on coal tar, or a water-based hair gel) will alleviate and may even solve both of these problem before you start applying the Acne Cure program. If the acne persists after you have made the modifications, it will disappear just as readily as acne vulgaris as soon as the Acne Cure program starts to take effect.

Acne Detergens

This occurs if you overwash your face. The solution is exceedingly simple: Don't! Instead (unless you work as a chimney sweep, garage mechanic, or construction worker, or in some other "dirty" job), clean your face with nothing but water for a few days.

Don't worry; your face won't become dirty. The sebum forms a layer between the dirt and the skin so that the dirt is barely attached to the surface, and the water rinses the loose dirt off easily enough.

You may be delighted to see that your acne has disappeared (along with the dirt) even before you start the program.

Acne Excoriee

This is the name given to a form of acne that is closer to a psychological than a skin condition. It is acne induced by an obsessive, sometimes self-abusive need to pick and squeeze even minute skin blemishes. In severe cases, patients may be distraught with their largely or wholly delusional conviction that their skin is "awful."

While, as with other "hysterical" reactions, eliminating the acne may in some cases help this condition to some degree, removal of the symptoms is not enough. Indeed, there is a condition called imaginary acne that results from the patients' conviction that they suffer from disfiguring acne when, in fact, they have few, if any, symptoms.

The cure of this condition, observed primarily in young women (and not infrequently associated with eating disorders, such as anorexia and bulimia), is difficult because the disease is not fully understood. If you know anyone who strongly expresses concern about her acne when you can see little trace of it, try to get her to see her doctor, and alert him or her that a psychiatrist or psychologist may be needed. You will not be betraying your friend (even if she told you in confidence); and, because acne excoriee is so often associated with potentially lethal eating disorders, you may be saving her life.

Acne Mallorca

This charmingly named form of the disease is caused directly by excess sunbathing, presumably of the type in which many people on that beautiful tourist island (called Majorca in English but Mallorca in Spanish and, presumably, in Latin) indulge. Sometimes it is mistaken for heat spots. Sometimes it is incorrectly diagnosed as a sun allergy. It apparently results from the heat of the sun causing more sebum production while, at the same time, more sweat swells the skin and thus tends to clog the pores that would allow its escape.

Regardless of what this type of acne is called, however, the cure is obvious and rapid: Remove yourself from the sun! (As you know, we firmly believe that this is sound strategy even if the sun is not immediately causing you to break out.)

Tropical Acne

Closely associated with acne mallorca is tropical acne. This affected our soldiers in Vietnam, sometimes grievously. Presumably it was caused by the excess sweat of a very hot and humid climate, coupled with both severe stress and the mechanical irritation of the skin caused by carrying weapons or other equipment (see acne mechanica, on the following page). Like all the other acnes in this list, it can be eradicated by the use of our Acne Cure protocol. However, to the extent that sufferers can spend at least part of each day in an air-conditioned environment, their acne will resolve itself that much more rapidly.

Acne Mechanica

As we have mentioned previously, the irritation and extra sweat caused by tight sports or work equipment may aggravate acne. However, the same equipment may be a necessary part of keeping fit or keeping your job. As such, our advice is continue to do what you have to do and solve the problem by the careful application of our Acne Cure program.

There is one often seen exception: Tight chin straps on helmets (wisely used for football, bike riding, and so on) sometimes cause rather severe localized acne where the straps touch the chin. Either you can avoid this problem by changing the straps' coverage area from time to time, or, if that is not feasible, you can largely eliminate the problem by placing a piece of absorbent lint between the strap and your skin. (If it won't stay in place, the lint can be held there with some surgical tape.) Once the strap no longer touches the skin directly, the acne in that location will almost always disappear.

Acne Medicamentosa

Several medications used for purposes unrelated to skin may cause or aggravate acne. However, the direct cause and effect between these drugs and the acne is not always clear; thus, it is important to confer with your doctor if you suspect that a drug you are taking may be impacting your acne.

The most common drugs that stand accused of exacerbating acne are:

• Dilantin (diphenylan sodium), used to treat grand mal seizures and prevent or treat seizures during and after brain surgery.

• Lithium, used to treat manic depression and, at lower dosages, to treat certain other psychological conditions, such as eating disorders and premenstrual tension.

• Micro-K and other comparable brands of potassium chloride, used to treat low potassium levels, particularly when a person is taking certain heart medications.

• Certain cold medications, especially those containing bromides or iodides. (Acne caused by these is characterized by very small pustules.)

• Various forms of birth control pills. As we have discussed previously, the impact of birth control pills on women's hormonal balance may boost sebum production and hence users' susceptibility to acne.

• Steroids. These may cause a distinctive form of acne beginning days or even weeks after the start of treatment. Steroid-induced acne appears as tiny red papules and pustules in the area to which the steroid was applied (if it was used topically) or on the chest, back, and shoulders (if the therapy was systemic). This form of acne occurs because the steroids tend to thin the dermis, making the follicular canals more likely to rupture inward. However, since the steroids are powerful anti-inflammatories, the lesions tend to be small. In some cases, they don't appear at all until after the drug use has been discontinued.

• In rare cases, other drugs, including actinomycin D, halothane, thiouracil, thiourea, trimethadiaone, and vitamin B_{12}.

In every case of acne medicamentosa, the first step is to check with your physician to see whether a change in medication is feasible. In many instances—as with steroids—even though no change is possible, the regimen is short-lived, and the problem will therefore quickly resolve itself. In others—as with birth control pills—there is a wide choice of appropriate alternatives. Although no one quite understands why, for some women making a change may stop the acne even though the new medication provides essentially the same hormones as the prior one, while for other women a change may have no effect at all.

If no medication change is feasible and the treatment is likely to continue for a long time or indefinitely—as with lithium—the probability is high that the standard acne cure protocol will nevertheless resolve the problem completely: The medication may have aggravated your acne, but it does not interfere with acne's elimination. However, if our treatment does not eradicate the disease completely, it must be treated as one of the more intractable versions.

Infant Acne

This condition, also called acne neonatorium, results from hormones passed from mother to fetus before birth and is not unusual. Generally, the condition cures itself within a few weeks after birth and requires no special treatment.

Sometimes the condition is relatively severe and not quickly resolved. In those cases, it is almost always eliminated by the application of the Acne Cure program.

However, a word of warning: Before using the Acne Cure on a newborn, please be certain to check with your pediatrician. While we believe that our program, judiciously applied, is safe even for the youngest infant, we want your physician to be sure that this applies to your particular baby. *Never* use the Acne Cure on your baby (or, for that matter, any cure for anything) without first checking with a doctor. With babies, one can never be too careful.

Chloracne

This is defined as acne induced by constant exposure to motor oil or insecticides.

We believe that if your exposure to these products is so severe and continuous as to induce acne, you are probably in danger of harming your health in more profound ways—for example, by overexposing your lungs to these toxins. Remember, we are not talking here about exposure to cooking oil such as you might experience in a Mc-Donald's kitchen. Rather, to induce chloracne, the degree of contamination has to be far worse than that. We therefore urge you to find a way to reduce the degree of contamination to which you are exposed. Doing so will largely eliminate your acne; the Acne Cure program will eradicate any remaining problem.

INTRACTABLE ACNES

Each of the above nine acnes (and variations of them) can be dealt with easily enough either by modifying their cause or by applying the Acne Cure—and certainly by a combination of both. That leaves four forms of acne that may in some cases require additional medical attention. They are acne conglobata, cystic acne, acne keloidalis nuchae (also called dermatitis papilaris capillitii), and acne fulminans.

There is also one other disease, called acne rosacea, that shows up, usually in women, as redness and bumps that look very much like acne. However, it is not acne at all, but a different skin condition. Because its genesis is quite different, it is not affected by either the basic Acne Cure or by the approaches to cure intractable acne discussed below.

The most important point to reemphasize about each of these forms of acne is that their development is exactly the same as that of acne vulgaris. The differences are merely ones of initial causation and severity.

For example, acne conglobata is a severe form of acne that tends to run in families and causes scarring on the face and back, sometimes to a considerable extent. It is especially common in people with an extra Y chromosome (XYY).

Cystic acne is differentiated only by the fact that a larger percentage of its comedones (compared with normal acne) rupture inward to cause the cysts we have described earlier.

Keloidal acne is largely confined to dark-skinned individuals. Once again, it is standard acne but of a type that unfortunately results in larger-than-normal numbers of keloids, particularly on the nape of the neck.

Acne fulminans is a particularly nasty, necrotic form of the disease where the cells in the area surrounding the acne cyst die out, leaving an unpleasant scar. It is accompanied by joint pain and even fever. Fortunately, it is quite rare.

There is no scientific explanation as to why some people fall victim to these more severe forms of acne. However, since all these forms of acne are caused by blockage of the follicular tubes, it follows that the severest cases occur when several different types of acne occur simultaneously—and aggravate one another. That is why, whatever type of acne you have, the first line of defense is to apply our Acne Cure program assiduously for a full 6 weeks. The result in many cases is nothing short of amazing.

In rarer cases, of course, while there has been a noticeable reduction in the severity of the disease, there has been no complete cure. In almost no case has Dr. Dubrow had a patient who showed no improvement while applying his cure. When no improvement occurred, the reason was inevitably that the patient had not applied the Acne Cure program correctly or completely.

CURING INTRACTABLE ACNE

We believe it is safe to say that even where the Acne Cure program fails to eliminate all acne symptoms, there are several other approaches that, added to this protocol, will eliminate virtually all the remaining symptoms. (We were tempted to write "eliminate all" rather than "eliminate virtually all" the symptoms, for that is in fact the case. We stopped ourselves only because, in medicine, there are no absolutes: However improbable, it is possible that somewhere someone has a case of acne that cannot be cured.)

Most cases of intractable acne will require the intervention of a physician since each involves the use of a prescription drug (in addition to applying Dr. Dubrow's program). Fortunately, the physician you consult will have a variety of options available to resolve your problem.

While the cure for the remaining intractable parts of your acne may vary according to the circumstances, the following is the four-step program that Dr. Dubrow recommends to most of his cure-re-sistant patients—and it works on (virtually) every one of them.

Step 1

Apply the basic Acne Cure program, exactly as described in chapter 4, for 4 weeks. If you see no improvement, you may have intractable acne. In that case, take careful notes of the skin's condition at that time (if possible, take photographs so that you have an accurate record). Now continue the program for another 2 weeks. If, after that time, there is further improvement, continue for yet another 2 weeks, and again reexamine the skin. Occasionally, you will continue to see improvement over several 2-week periods; the Cure is working, but more slowly than usual. Continue to apply the full program in 2-week increments until there is no further improvement over the last 2 weeks.

Step 2

While continuing the treatment, add an intensive Retin-A treatment, increasing frequency over a 3-week period as follows:

Your doctor will prescribe the concentration of Retin-A that is most appropriate for your skin, and will advise you on how to use it to best effect. Generally, we recommend that you apply it in the evening before your final ice and BP treatment.

You can expect to see some redness as you implement this plan, usually during the second week. However, if it starts to become severe, or if you start to suffer from unpleasant irritation, reduce the frequency.

Step 3

If the acne persists beyond the 3-week period of Retin-A usage, continue the Acne Cure program, but stop the Retin-A. Instead, add an internally administered antibiotic.

Tetracycline, that old but effective standby, works well for most patients—and is relatively inexpensive and widely used. Several other antibiotics also work well (although all have possible side effects). Your physician, knowing your history, will advise you of your best alternative, dosage, and length of usage.

Tetracycline and minocyclin (and several other antibiotics), in addition to destroying *P. acnes*, have an anti-inflammatory impact, which helps slow down the spread of the disease.

Step 4

Very rarely indeed does anyone have to progress as far as Step 4. However, if some *continuing* acne remains, the final step is to take Accutane. We have noted earlier the dangers associated with this drug. It is worth repeating, however, that Accutane should never be taken by pregnant women or those who may become pregnant.

We stress "continuing" because sometimes, after the acne has actually been eliminated, one or two severe lesions remain. These may have become infected, have formed closed cysts, or otherwise remain "uncured." However, their continued presence doesn't necessarily mean that the disease remains. Thus, rather than start you on Accutane, your physician will probably want to deal with such lesions individually, usually by the injection into them of a corticosteroid and occasionally by surgical excision.

There are many other acne medications, ranging from "natural" products such as primrose oil (which we think has no positive effect on acne) to a European medication called cyproterone acetate. However, in our view none of these products, even if somewhat effective, is needed. The Acne Cure program will eradicate the large majority of acne, and the remainder will be entirely wiped out by one or more of the steps in the four-step "intractable acne" program described above.

As we have said before, there is no need for anyone to suffer from the physical or psychological distress of even the most severe continuing acne.

Unfortunately, however, if you have had acne in the past and it has left you with unsightly scarring, you may be facing a separate problem. While your acne was active, your main concern was naturally to cure it. Once that objective was accomplished, you might have decided that the time was ripe to resolve the aftermath of that earlier acne, the pits and pocks of the disease that was not cured soon enough. The next chapter will deal with how to minimize that problem.

12

ELIMINATING ACNE SCARS

NOT EVERYONE WORRIES about residual acne scars. Particularly in men, the impression an acne-pitted face makes may be of virility rather than ugliness. We know of several successful film stars whose faces carry dramatically visible acne scars and who apparently do nothing to hide them—Edward James Olmos and Tommy Lee Jones come to mind. Perhaps too, they and others like them adhere to the philosophy of one Anthony Euwer, an early-20th-century writer of rhymes and limericks, who claimed:

There are others more handsome by far

But my face—I don't mind it

For I am behind it.

It's the people in front get the jar.

On the other hand, like it or not, even in today's society of equality, women's skin is viewed by them (and by the men who love and cherish them) as one of their special features. Or, as Alfred, Lord Tennyson, put it:

Man is the hunter; woman is the game:

The sleek and shining creatures of the chase,

We hunt them for the beauty of their skins.

No one wants that beauty marred by the pits and scarring of past acne. And, happily, there is a great deal we can now do to rectify the problem. In the worst cases, scarring cannot be entirely eliminated, but it can be reduced to the point where in women makeup can completely hide any remaining problems, and in men the remaining scars are rarely considered to be seriously unsightly.

WHAT CAUSES SCARRING?

To understand what can be done about residual acne scars, we must first understand why scars form in the first place.

Obviously, scars are the aftermath of the body's skin-healing process. This is an ongoing process that starts the moment the wound is formed and continues for at least a year—sometimes longer—until the scar is both formed and then minimized.

The first step in the scarring process is that the open wound (or acne lesion, now cured of its infection but still open and raw) becomes inflamed. That is to say, blood rushes in, carrying a whole pharmacopoeia of specialized chemicals. (Even when we use anti-inflammatories, or we reduce the speed of the blood inflow with ice packs, blood remains essential to the curative process.) The ingredients that blood carries to the scene include:

- Chemicals that diminish bloodflow by constricting damaged blood vessels. If this did not happen, your acne wounds would continue to bleed.

- Platelets to plug up any remaining leaks.

• White corpuscles to fight off any bacteria from the skin's surface that would normally be held off by intact skin.

The second stage in the healing (and, unintentionally, scarring) process is that the acne wounds start to fill up with a material called granulation tissue. As this happens, the wounds also start to contract as specialized cells generate new collagen. As the collagen generates, the epidermis starts to grow over the granulation tissue, leaving the skin over the wound very similar to (and often indistinguishable from) the surrounding skin in both consistency and color. Even so, some scar tissue remains, and the body deals with this very slowly as an enzyme called collagenase gradually eats away at any excess scar tissue and so remodels the scar until it is largely invisible.

Unfortunately, even when this process is complete—which may take up to a year—several types of acne scars may remain, specifically:

• **"Ice pick" scars.** These are small (about 1 to 2 millimeters in diameter), deep scars with sharp edges that look as if a tiny cookie cutter had punched them out. They are generally the aftermath of acne that has penetrated deep into the skin—cystic acne is the most common culprit—so that the wound caused by the acne extends from the skin's surface to the base of the dermis. What happens is that a vertical band of collagen forms along the full length of the "wounded" follicular tube. In repairing the wound, this collagen "rope," anchored at the bottom of the dermis, contracts and pulls down the surface of the skin into a deep and well-defined "pock."

• **Pitted scars.** These are more shallow impressions than the deep ice pick pockmarks, but they may be wider, sometimes as much as half the diameter of a dime. They are the result of acne that penetrated less deeply and therefore healed more rapidly. Because of this speedy recovery (or perhaps for a variety of other reasons), the body didn't produce quite enough granulation tissue to avoid a depression on the surface of the skin.

• **Hypertrophic scarring.** This occurs when the body overproduces fresh scar tissue, which then shows up as a tiny raised "welt," or bump, on the skin's surface. It happens more frequently with wounds other than those from acne, but it may apply to acne as well. Moreover, since it happens more frequently in young than in older people, there is a reasonable chance that this type of scarring in adults may be the remaining reminder of severe teenage acne. (We suspect that one reason adults so dislike acne scars is that they are a constant reminder of the "awful" trauma their acne caused them when they were teenagers.)

Over time, hypertrophic scars gradually become less visible as the collagenase enzyme eats away at the excess scar tissue. However, although sometimes that process continues until no scars remain, at other times a degree of residual scarring never does disappear completely.

• **Keloids.** These are a particular problem for Black skin. More rarely, they also occur in other races when there happens to be a genetic predisposition for their formation.

Keloids are darkened, thick, raised tumors caused by a genetic condition that influences the body to overproduce scar tissue. Thus, for reasons we do not understand, in some people the fibroblasts that produce the collagen needed to heal the wound do not stop the production of the scar tissue soon enough—and keloids result. Unfortunately, unlike hypertrophic scars, keloids don't shrink over time. Moreover, in addition to being raised, black or dark brown, and rough, they may itch and cause pain or irritation. Consequently—even though they rarely appear on the face, limiting their aggression to the chest, shoulders, upper back, neck, and (strangely) the earlobes—in most cases they have to be removed. (The susceptibility of the earlobes to keloids is one reason that people, especially people of color, who wish to have their ears pierced should have it done under rigorously sterile conditions, preferably in a doctor's office, rather than in some jewelry shop.)

• **Discoloration.** Strictly speaking, discoloration—which may take the form of redness on White skin or darker spots on dark skin—is not scarring. However, it may be just as unsightly.

The red spots on light-colored skin are the result of extra blood vessels that have formed in the area in order to cure the acne-caused infections. In nearly all cases, these extra blood vessels will gradually be reabsorbed once the infection is gone and the extra blood is no longer needed.

On the other hand, the dark spots visible in darker-skinned people are caused by the stimulation of the pigment-producing cells. Since the extra pigment lodges deep inside the dermis, it may remain there for a very long time, even permanently.

There is also a condition, called a fixed drug eruption, that is applicable only to dark-skinned people. Brought on by certain medications, fixed drug eruption shows up as harmless but unsightly black discolorations that may continue for months or even permanently and that worsen with each exposure to the medication.

Fixed drug eruptions may result from taking various medications, including some—such as ampicillin and tetracycline—used to combat unusually resistant forms of acne. If you are dark-skinned and your doctor prescribes drugs for your acne, be sure to inquire as to whether there is any danger of their causing fixed drug eruptions. If he or she is not aware of the problem, we suggest you visit a different physician.

In discussing these five forms of scarring, we should emphasize that they are not necessarily clearly differentiated. In practice, people with substantial visible scarring are likely to have a combination of several different sorts of acne scars. Each person's case is different, and each must be evaluated individually.

THE ACNE CURE
SCAR REMOVAL PROCESS

Acne scarring can be treated and greatly improved. However, no complete resolution is possible in the worst cases. Thus, patients who are upset about the appearance of their skin should be made aware, before they start the process of eliminating their scars, that even the most sophisticated treatment—and the most skilled of plastic surgeons—may not be able to return their skin to its pristine, pre-acne condition.

We should further emphasize that the removal of scars may take a considerable amount of time. That is because most of the treatments involve first "damaging" the skin, or removing its surface, and then allowing it to repair and rejuvenate itself with less scarring. This naturally takes time.

Finally, before proceeding to describe scarring treatments, we should add three caveats:

1. Before you deal with old scars, make sure your current acne is fully cured. Most treatments for scarring represent an assault on the skin. You don't want to undertake such an assault while new acne still lurks, ready to join the attack.

2. Since collagenase can take a long time to dissolve excess scar tissue, wait at least a year after your last acne attack before doing anything about the remaining scars. Even then, check carefully over the last 2 months (again, keeping a photographic record, if possible) to see whether the scarring is improving. As long as some improvement continues, don't do anything; you may be doing yourself more harm than good. Once the scar "reorganization" process is complete, you may find that the problem you were so worried about has largely or entirely cured itself.

3. Waiting a year is especially important if you are one of the few people forced to take Accutane to eliminate the residual acne left after completion of the Acne Cure program. That is because there is some evidence that, after using Accutane, patients are more likely to experience undesirable scarring after any skin damage. So play it safe!

Given the fact that scar removal by any technique may not be perfect and, in any case, is likely to take a long time, we recommend a step-by-step approach to resolve the problem. Each step escalates the vigor of your scar attack. That way, at the end of each step, you can evaluate whether you feel the problem has now receded sufficiently or it is worth proceeding to the next, more aggressive (and generally more painful and expensive) step.

Of course, this "step" process is only a general recommendation. Since each step must be carried out under the supervision of (and often by) a qualified physician, his or her advice must always be determinant.

The step process Dr. Dubrow generally recommends to his patients is as follows.

Step 1: Bleach

This step applies particularly if you suffer from hyperpigmentation. To eradicate, or at least greatly lessen, your dark spots, first implement the 3-week Retin-A program outlined in chapter 11 as a step in dealing with intractable acne. Once the intensive part of that effort is complete, use a topical hydroquinine cream (also sold as bleaching cream) to further fade the dark spots. And throughout, be doubly careful to avoid sun.

Bleaching cream is available over-the-counter at a 2% strength. Start with this, and apply it once a day in the morning (apply the Retin-A in the evening). Continue for 3 weeks. If you note an improvement, continue for 2-week periods until you see no further progress. The same product is available by prescription at a 4% strength. If the weaker strength is not working, we suggest that (subject to your doctor's concurrence, of course) you move to the stronger version.

While this step is especially appropriate to deal with hyperpigmentation, the combination of these two relatively mild treatments is often surprisingly effective in reducing the visibility of acne scars.

Step 2: Apply a Chemical Peel

There are three levels of peel. The mildest form is to use our old friend glycolic acid at a concentration—up to 35%—that does not require a prescription and can therefore be used by an aesthetician. The glycolic acid is applied for a period of time to the skin, then neutralized with a mild alkali, and washed off with water. This type of peel may help to some extent, but at these relatively low concentrations, you should not expect much effect.

Two other types of chemical peels are sometimes applied:

1. A "medium" peel, using either trichloracetic acid, a similar commercial product called Jessener's Solution, or glycolic acid at a

concentration of 50 to 70%. Often physicians recommend that, after they have conducted the glycolic acid peel, the patient complete the procedure at home, using a 20 to 30% glycolic acid gel daily for the next 7 to 14 days.

2. A "deep" phenol peel (sometimes using a commercial product known as Baker's Solution).

In general, we believe that when it comes to chemical peels, neither extreme is desirable. That is to say, a glycolic acid peel performed at a concentration of less than 50% is likely to have only limited success. And phenol peels—designed to do as much "damage" as dermabrasion, or more—seem to us to be more dangerous without doing more good. Indeed, phenol may be harmful to the heart, and we recommend against its use.

Thus, on balance, we recommend using a 50 to 70% glycolic acid peel under the supervision of a physician.

Whatever form of chemical peel is used, if it is successful, the skin first forms a sort of mask, which then peels off. If you see a significant improvement from the chemical peel, we suggest you repeat it after about a month. You can do this several times. However, once you see no further improvement, and assuming you are not yet satisfied, wait at least a month before proceeding to Step 3.

Step 3: Dermabrasion

This involves removing the top layer of the skin down to the upper surface of the dermis. In the past it was done by mechanical means; a small diamond burr was used to scrape off the top layer of skin.

The difficulty with this approach is that it may leave fair skin very red for weeks or even for several months, and it may cause dark skin to darken unevenly; the resulting mottled appearance can become permanent.

Fortunately, the positive effects of dermabrasion can now be achieved by the use of a laser. This technique, pioneered in the early 1990s by California physician Richard Fitzpatrick, M.D., and others, uses the energy of carbon dioxide (CO_2) to strip off the top layer of skin. More recently, a new form of laser called a YAG laser has further improved the technique by allowing for a finer layer of skin to be removed. This requires more passes over certain parts of the skin but also gives the administering dermatologist or plastic surgeon more control and causes less damage to the surrounding tissue. This means there is generally a lot less redness and much quicker healing.

Both forms of laser generate invisible infrared light, which rapidly vaporizes the water in your skin cells. In doing so, the light "burns off" anywhere from 20 to 100 microns of skin—nearer the lower thickness for YAG lasers, closer to the greater thickness for CO_2 lasers. (For comparison, a sheet of paper is about 100 microns thick.)

There is no doubt that in many cases, removing a layer of skin by dermabrasion or (preferably) by laser treatment will reduce scarring. However, the treatment may have to be repeated several times at intervals of at least 2 months to become as effective as possible. Even then, deep ice pick scars will likely remain, and the surface of your skin will not be perfect. If you don't have overoptimistic expectations, you will not be disappointed. Step 3 of scar removal will almost always show a significant improvement.

Step 4: Remove Major Scars, Keloids, and Similar Blemishes

There are three basic ways in which this can be achieved.

1. Flat scars can be filled in by injecting collagen under them, thus pushing them up to the same level as the rest of the skin. This technique is relatively quick and simple. However, it lasts only a few months, as the body gradually absorbs the collagen. Most people find that to maintain essentially scar-free complexions, they have to repeat the procedure about twice a year.

Rarely, a patient experiences an allergic reaction to collagen injections; in that case, the procedure obviously cannot be used.

2. Ice pick scarring may necessitate a more extreme removal system. Since the scars are anchored to the bottom layer of the skin, in many cases the collagen injections will not push them out, or at least not far enough. Where this is the case, the doctor, after anesthetizing the area, will cut out the pock—with a device that looks like a small cookie cutter and can be adjusted to be just barely larger than the pock—and then sew the skin together with tiny sutures. When the wounds heal, the remaining scars will be barely visible. In addition, they can then be almost completely smoothed away and made quite invisible by a subsequent overall laser treatment.

As with any surgical procedure, there is some risk to this approach. However, performed by a competent and experienced physician, the risk is minimal.

3. Keloids (whether caused by acne or other conditions) are the most difficult blemishes to remove not the least because they have a tendency to re-form. Moreover, even though they may not be in a particularly visible location, they generally must be removed because they become irritated—and often continue to grow. Sometimes, they can be halted in their tracks by the injection of Kenalog (or another triamcinolone). If that doesn't work, surgical excision is needed, ideally followed by localized radiation therapy to inhibit the activity of the fibroblasts and thus stop the keloids from re-forming.

CONCLUSION

It goes without saying that the best way to deal with acne scarring is to avoid it in the first place. And, having read this far, you know that you need never worry about future scarring. However, if you have scars from past acne, there is no point in saying they could have been avoided. That is about as useful as an author in one book we ran across who explained with great authority that "to prevent hypertrophic scarring, avoid injury to the skin." How could you disagree with that?

Fortunately, when it comes to acne-generated scarring, there is a lot you can do.

In all likelihood, the removal of your current acne, coupled with Step 1 of our anti-scar program—that is, 3 weeks of intense Retin-A treatment, followed by the use of a bleaching cream—will make your complexion look so much better that you may decide that further treatment is unnecessary.

If that is not the case, the subsequent three steps as outlined on the preceding pages (under the close supervision of your physician) will solve most of the problem. Whatever your age, you will look healthier, more rested, and altogether more attractive. And if you are over 35, you will find that many of your fine wrinkles will also disappear. You will look younger—and, unless we miss our bet, you will feel terrific!

No more acne; far fewer, less visible scars; and a healthier, more glowing and "awake" complexion. Even if some acne scars remain—milder and less visible, to be sure—you will no longer have much wrong with your looks, and certainly nothing to be concerned about. As a matter of fact, you will look great!

13

ACNE MYTHS
AND OLD WIVES' TALES

OLD WIVES' TALES ARE FASCINATING because even when they are clearly wrong, they often contain a grain of truth—or at least a grain of rather perverse logic—which seems to make them plausible . . . and therefore even more thoroughly wrong!

To cite just one example, take the well-known "fact" that cranberry juice is good for kidney and urinary tract problems. The truth is that, medically, cranberry juice is no better or worse than orange juice. However, it is a far less universally popular a taste, and it tends to cost more. Reasonably, then, one would expect that orange would be the juice of choice. Nevertheless, virtually all nurses and hospital administrators— and quite a few urologists—specify cranberry juice, sincerely believing it to be better for their patients. But why, when it is not?

The answer probably lies in a long-known but largely forgotten fact, namely that cranberry juice (unlike orange or any other fruit juice) has the unique property of deodorizing urine . . . which, of course, makes nurses' cleanup task a lot pleasanter. Over the years, that correct fact appears to have been transmogrified into "cranberry juice is better"!

Similarly, any number of old wives' tales surrounding acne, while wrong, have a foundation of a correct but misinterpreted fact. Let us consider the most widely circulated of these tales and identify whether they are true or false and, if false, how they gained their currency.

GENERAL MYTHS ABOUT ACNE

There are three sorts of myths about acne: those that deal with puta-
tive causes, those that deal with supposed cures, and those that deal
with the conditions surrounding the disease. Since the last are the
least diverse, let us deal with them first.

Really Severe Acne Is Catching

Many skin diseases are indeed highly contagious. Acne is not one of
them. Since *P. acnes* bacteria exist on all human skin, there is nothing
that surface contact will transmit from one person to another that is
not already there.

Conceivably, if acne is left untreated, becomes very severe, and
then leads to a really nasty secondary infection, *that* might possibly
be transmitted to another person who also has open, but not yet infected, lesions. However, this circumstance is far-fetched—there is no
need for things ever to get that out of hand. As a general rule, acne is
not contagious.

Infant Acne Always Leads to Teenage Acne

This is not true. There appears to be no correlation between ordi-
nary infant acne and teenage acne. However, since most teenagers
do suffer from acne, it is true that most babies who experience infant acne will also develop the teenage form. But, then, so will the
majority of teenagers who never showed symptoms of the disease as
newborns.

However, the situation here is even a little more confused because
there is one form of infant acne that is hereditary, usually from the father. Left untreated, it would persist for months or years in the infant
and would be very likely to recur in the teenager.

Thus, this old wives' tales has some basis in fact—even though it is not generally true.

Acne and Balding Are Related

Male-type hormones, or androgens, affect both hair and oil glands, tending to speed up the loss of one and the production of the other. Thus, theoretically, bald men may be more likely to suffer from acne. However, if there is any truth to this rumor, it has yet to be proven, a task complicated by the fact that acne tends to decrease and baldness obviously tends to increase with age. On balance, we believe that there is no significant likelihood that if you are a man, you will be cursed with premature balding and long-lasting acne at the same time. One scourge at a time!

The situation is slightly different for women. There is a rare condition where women, whose ovaries normally produce low levels of androgens, overproduce the hormones. This may lead to a number of symptoms, including increased facial hair, a loss of scalp hair, and acne, sometimes severe. The appearance of any such symptoms necessitates immediate medical intervention.

Acne Scars Get Worse with Age

No, this is not true. However, here is another situation where the "untrue" old wives' tale has a grain of truth buried within it.

What actually happens as we age is that the loss of elastin tissue combined with the weakening of the muscles causes various "sags" to appear. Sometimes these sags pull one or more acne scars out of shape—so that they look larger or more pronounced than they did originally.

So . . . acne scars don't actually get worse as we age—but sometimes they look worse!

MYTHICAL CAUSES OF ACNE

There are "facts" that we heard at our mother's knee that they "knew" to be true with absolute, total, unassailable conviction. Wet feet and drafts cause colds. Wine gets better when it breathes. Arthritis acting up predicts a brewing storm. All these are false. But not necessarily completely false. And the same applies to the myths about what causes acne. False, false, but not necessarily completely so . . .

Poor Hygiene Causes Acne—So Wash Your Face!

This is probably the mother of all myths—fostered, no doubt, by all old wives' conviction that youngsters are inherently dirty, that cleanliness is next to godliness, that dirt is therefore the work of the devil, and that acne is the punishment for such work.

"Slovenliness is no part of religion," preached John Wesley, co-founder of the Methodist religion.

"Wash your mouth out," our mothers used to remonstrate. "And while you're at it, wash your face."

No doubt, looking thoroughly scrubbed and clean has its advantages. However, with respect to acne, excessive washing is a bad idea for the reasons we have elucidated earlier. Nor is a dirty face, however undesirable it may be for aesthetic reasons, going to cause acne.

By all means wash your face. But do so with plain water if that is enough to loosen the surface dirt. If it takes more than that, use the mildest cleanser you can find. Reserve the more thorough washings for those of your body interstices that are likely to cause unpleasant body odor—and unlikely to develop acne.

Masturbation Exacerbates Acne

The myth that masturbation causes or at least exacerbates acne is a tenacious one. According to Peter Engel, coauthor of a book called

Old Wives' Tales, these sorts of myths about the dangers of mastur-bation "started as a warning from parents in the [19th] century to stop their male children from committing the 'self-polluting act.' Incipient insanity, epilepsy, weakened physique, shifty eyes, and hairy palms were . . . threatened consequences of what was referred to as 'self-abuse.' "[1] Just as those results were wholly false, so is the persistent belief that masturbation has any impact on acne. There is no need to control masturbation (and thus acne), as did the Victorians, by inserting spikes under boys' foreskins!

However, in addition to the aftermath of the baseless tradition that masturbation is generally bad for you, with respect to acne the belief gains plausibility because, while there is no cause-and-effect relationship between masturbation and acne, there is certainly a correlation between them. The hormonal changes that occur at the start of puberty lead to several concurrent phenomena. One of these is that, in many youngsters, they give rise to acne. And, of course, this is also the time nearly all boys and the large majority of girls start to masturbate. Not surprisingly, some think the acne is the result of (or perhaps the punishment for) the masturbation. It isn't.

Your First Shave Will Give You Acne

Puberty is also the time that boys experience the first sign of a beard. Initially, the hair on a young man's face is sparse—the "fuzz" you see on the chins of teenage boys, of which they are often inordinately proud. With the passage of time, these beards become denser and thicker. But long before that happens, as often as not, the young man, striving for manliness, starts to shave. Since the new hair that follows the shave grows in thicker, the youth naturally assumes that it was the shaving that did it (just as pruning the top off a plant often makes its stem thicker). An old wives' tale—wholly incorrect—is born.

Shaving has no impact on the density or thickness of hair, but the young man, unaware of his misobservation, continues to shave, more often and more vigorously than necessary. The result is that he dries out his skin and, in cutting the hairs to below its surface, encourages them to turn on themselves and grow inward, causing pimples that (as we explained earlier) look much like acne. Both of these phenomena, coupled with the hormones that encourage sebum production, may cause acne (and pseudo-acne) to be more frequent, earlier, and more severe than it would otherwise be.

So, no, first shaving—or any other shaving, for that matter—does not cause acne; but teenage boys' shaving too often and too close may contribute to it.

Eating Chocolate Causes Acne

In our still (at least distantly) Puritan society, all pleasures, certainly including masturbation and chocolate, are prone to be considered somehow "wicked," or at least so self-indulgent that they are bound to lead to some sort of punishment. In the case of chocolate, the punishment, as "everyone knows," is that it causes acne.

This is wrong. In their book *Skin Deep*, Drs. Turkington and Dover wrote, "In one study, 65 people ate chocolate bars every day for a month, but although the bars contained 10 times the normal amount of chocolate, the subjects experienced no worsening of blemishes."[2] And researchers at the University of Pennsylvania fed 50 teenagers with acne a pound of chocolate a day. The result was that the acne of 46 of them remained unchanged; two got worse; and two got better.[3] (There is no mention in this research of the impact of the intake of a pound of chocolate a day on any other aspect of the teenagers' health, but we do not recommend it!)

The fact is, there is nothing in chocolate that has any direct effect on acne.

However, this is where the magic of correlation, that is two things happening at the same time but not related to each other, rears its head. Over and over again, we all seem to make the mistake of assuming that where there is a clear correlation, there must be a cause and a direct effect.

For example, in a study conducted in the 1970s by the Helena Rubinstein cosmetic company, researchers found that when they changed the package but not the content of one skin treatment cream, between 10 and 20 percent of its purchasers felt that the "new" product caused their skin to break out. This finding is in line with the experience of most industry experts. The reason is that at any moment, between 10 and 20 percent of women suffer from a new outbreak of some form of acne, minor skin rash, or blemish. When that happens routinely, the women ignore it, ascribing it to their menstrual cycles, something they ate, or perhaps to a particularly stressful event. But if, immediately before the breakout, they used a "new" cosmetic cream, it is that product that gets the blame. A correlation is seen as a causative event.

Taken to an extreme, you can find some strange facts that are "proven" by correlations. For example, for many years there was a statistically significant correlation between the number of babies born in Holland and the number of storks in that country. See, we told you so!

In the case of chocolate eating, there are three correlations that may play a role in fostering the erroneous belief that the confection leads to acne.

1. Teenagers are renowned for going on chocolate eating "binges" (chocolate cake, chocolate ice cream, chocolate anything). At the same time, they often suffer from outbreaks of acne. If one of those outbreaks follows hard on the heels of a chocolate binge, the timing coincidence (coupled with the youngster's guilt at having downed

10 Hershey bars in a row) leads to the certainty that the chocolate caused the zits.

2. At a more general level, people who overindulge in chocolate are less likely to be on a healthy, antioxidant-rich diet. As a result of insufficient antioxidants, they may well be more subject to acne attacks. It's not the chocolate that does it; it's an overall poor diet, of which excessive chocolate consumption may be just one symptom.

3. Finally, people who eat a lot of chocolate and who, coincidentally, also subsist on a bad diet (possibly including Dunkin' Donuts, double cheeseburgers, french fries, and beer) may become fat. If that excess weight and girth leads to tight clothing and extra sweat, it may also lead to more acne. But again, the correlation proves nothing. Chocolate is an innocent contributor to a much more general problem.

Oily Foods Cause Acne

Nuts, butter, oil, cheese, peanut butter, french fries, fried chicken— and probably many other greasy foods—have all, at one time or another, been blamed for causing zits. Abstaining from these foods is, once again, "well-known" to help clear up your skin.

And, once again, the information is no more correct for oils and fats than it is for chocolate. If such foods are part of a generally unhealthy diet, they are bad for you—and for your skin. If they are consumed only in moderation, and only occasionally—or if they are counteracted with sufficient exercise and complemented with an otherwise healthy diet—they will not cause, worsen, or in any way affect acne.

Other Foods Cause Acne

Many different foods have been blamed for causing or aggravating acne. Shellfish, sugar, mushrooms, tomatoes, and who knows what other foods have at times been seen as causing acne. But the fact is that the foods you eat have no impact on your acne—except in the general sense that the good diet improves your overall health, and good health, including good skin health, will tend to mitigate the negative impact of acne.

However, there is one diet ingredient that has been shown to have a meaningful, direct and negative impact on acne. Dietary iodides are excreted through the sebum-producing sebaceous glands and may cause an acne flare-up, usually within 10 to 15 days of the start of consumption. Such iodides are not widely available. However, they are occasionally found in three sources. Two of them—certain dietary supplements and some seaweeds—are rare and it is unlikely that you would be consuming large quantities of them, although it is not impossible if you have started on one of several rather exotic diets.

More probable is the third source of iodide: It is found in certain water supplies, especially in the Caribbean islands, where the drinking water is desalinized seawater. If your acne broke out a few days after you started your Caribbean vacation, it may be the result of iodide in the drinking water. Of course, if the acne starts about the time you are returning, it may be the result of the stress caused by the overloaded in basket you face on getting back to your office. If the acne disappears spontaneously within a few days, chances are it was the drinking water. If it doesn't, stress may be the culprit. In either case, of course, the treatment program we have described can eliminate the problem.

Allergies Cause Acne

Contrary to popular belief, although allergic reactions to the environment and to the foods you eat are a frequent problem for many people, such reactions to other manufactured products you consume are rare. For example, only about three out of every thousand prescriptions written cause an allergic reaction.

Adverse drug reactions are more frequent; a breakout due to such a reaction is called an exanthem. For example, tetracycline and some other antibiotics will occasionally cause a reddening of the skin that may look like the start of acne. It isn't, and it will go away either spontaneously while you are still on the medication, or definitely within a day or two after you stop.

Similarly, almost no cosmetics cause an allergic reaction. Both the individual ingredients and the formulated products are exhaustively tested, first on animals and then on humans. (By the way, even those companies that boast that they do no animal testing on their products usually buy only ingredients that others once tested on animals.) Once a new ingredient has been carefully tested, both on animals and on humans, its manufacturer usually defrays the cost of doing so by selling it to many different companies. They in turn, pleased with a new and presumably improved product, incorporate it into many different brands, which are then sold over the years to millions and millions of people. Any product or ingredient that caused any noticeable level of allergic reaction would be promptly withdrawn from the market. Not only would its manufacturers be far too frightened of being sued to continue to sell it, but to do so would be unnecessary. Why sell an allergenic product when there are so many nonallergenic ones available?

No, there is very little chance that you will suffer from an allergic reaction to a medication, and virtually none that you will have such a reaction to a cosmetic. But even if you did, that reaction would not cause acne.

Having said that, as we have stressed elsewhere, cosmetic products that are greasy and occlude the skin do help to form the comedones that cause acne. Always use oil-free moisturizers.

Waxing Causes Acne

Removing hairs by painting on melted wax, letting it harden around the hairs, and then stripping it off—often practiced by women on their legs, arms, or bikini areas—may cause folliculitis, an infection of the hair follicles. However, this is an infection by staphylococcus bacteria, not by *P. acnes*. It has nothing to do with acne. It is cured by a course of an appropriate antibiotic.

It is true that certain types of folliculitis form small red pustules, sometimes with tiny heads of pus. Thus, they look very much like acne. Moreover, since these pimples obviously appear in the same place as acne—that is, at the mouth of the follicular tube—they can sometimes be misdiagnosed as acne. However, this is a simple case of mistaken identity. Waxing does not cause acne.

MYTHICAL CURES

Just as there are countless "well-known" but totally incorrect "causes" for acne, so there are countless equally accepted "cures." They too are nearly all wrong. Let us touch on just a few.

Camphor Is a Sure Cure for Acne

Camphor is a volatile compound derived from an Asian evergreen tree. It is used in some cosmetic compounds because it makes the skin feel warm, and it helps to relieve itching to some extent because it has a slight numbing effect.

Camphor is touted by many aestheticians and so-called skin specialists (who are not, however, physicians) as a product that can quickly alleviate sudden skin outbreaks. "A camphor mask will work wonders," they will assure the unsuspecting beauty parlor client. And sometimes it works—but no more often than doing nothing!

The truth is that camphor does nothing for any known skin rash or for acne. The best that can be said for it is that it does no known harm.

Sun Exposure Cures Acne

As we have stressed throughout this book, unprotected sun exposure is bad for your skin. In addition to the long-term damage it undoubtedly does, leading to a higher risk of skin cancer and inevitably to earlier, more severe wrinkling, sun can dry the stratum corneum and thus give rise to increased flaking—and an increased probability of clogged pores and hence acne.

In addition, sun exposure can also cause or aggravate certain drug-related reactions. For example, if you take sulfa drugs, anti-inflammatory drugs such as piroxicam, certain members of the tetracycline family, St. John's wort, and a common antifungal product called grisefulvin, those chemicals are distributed throughout your body, including in your skin. Then, when too much ultraviolet light falls on the skin's surface, it may react with the chemicals to cause a rash. Clearly, this is not acne, but it can cause redness and itching. The answer, of course, is to use a sunblock if you are on any medication—and even if you are not!

By all means, go into the sun. But make certain you always use a sunblock—and reapply it often enough if the sunlight is strong and direct. Wearing a hat on especially sunny days is a pretty good idea too. The sun will not cure your acne, but by protecting your skin from ultraviolet light damage, you will help it remain healthier and wrinkle-free. In the long run, you may even make it more resistant to acne.

Alcohol Dries Away Acne

This myth applies to vodka that, applied to the skin, will dry away your acne in no time. Or so the old wives assure us.

But, as we have stressed before, this is very wrong indeed. Alcohol will, on occasion, reduce the secondary infection from an open wound. But acne is a very different matter.

The only way that alcohol might help acne (provided its use is sensibly controlled) is by letting you relax happily over a cocktail after a tough day at the office. A nice, cold martini may lessen stress, and less stress may inhibit acne. The poet Robert Browning explained that a "stiffish cocktail, taken in time, is better for a bruise than arnica." He might have added that, similarly taken in time, it can also work wonders for stress-induced acne!

So never apply that alcohol to your skin's surface. If you do, it will certainly dry things up and thus generate more dry skin cells. But the sebum emerging from your pores will continue unabated. The result, after the first few minutes, will be that clogs are more, not less, likely to form and lead to acne.

Don't use alcohol or alcohol-based products on your skin.

Essential Oils Help Cure Acne

Several essential oils—in particular lavender, lemon, rosemary, sage, tea tree, and thyme—have been touted as being helpful to blemished skin. Indeed, as Myriam Zaoui and Eric Malka pointed out in their book *The Art of Shaving*, "The practice of using essential oils for medicinal and cosmetic purposes is at least 6,000 years old. . . . From the ancient Egyptians to the Greeks, Romans, Arabs, Chinese, and North American Indians, essential oils have been used for . . . their therapeutic characteristics."[4]

How can one argue with such a lengthy pedigree—except, perhaps, to point out that for virtually that entire time, the medicine practiced by those ancients commonly resulted in a life expectancy less than half of what we enjoy today? Notwithstanding this obvious fact, old wives' tales seem to gain vigor with age.

Perhaps essential oils have some therapeutic value. Certainly, advocates of aromatherapy swear by them. However, they do nothing for acne!

CONCLUSION

The Acne Cure program we have outlined in chapter 4 is an effective cure for the vast majority of cases of acne. The remaining, more intractable cases can also be cured, by the techniques we discussed in chapter 11. And acne scars left from earlier, untreated acne can be largely eliminated by the methods outlined in chapter 12.

Thus, usually for very little money and in no more than 6 weeks, your acne can be eradicated once and for all. There is no need for any of the mythological cures the old wives advocate. Which is just as well, because they don't work!

14

CONCLUSION

ACNE IS GENETIC. Thus, when both parents suffered from acne, three out of four of their children are likely to share the problem. That is because acne is a dominant gene. Moreover, even the type of acne and its location on the face, chest, neck, or back is genetically predisposed. For example, if a father's acne was severe but largely confined to the chest, quite often the children will suffer from the same condition in the same location.

So, as with many conditions, you are more or less likely to have severe acne according to the coincidence of your birth. Fortunately, as we have explained, the fact that you are *prone* to acne as a result of your genetics doesn't mean that you have to *have* acne. It means only that you are prone to suffer from a curable disease. If that is the most negative inherited factor with which you are burdened, you're in pretty good shape.

The problem is that, although acne can be almost entirely eradicated with a simple, inexpensive treatment (as we have emphasized throughout this book), more often than not, an inherited tendency toward getting acne results in an unsightly, painful, and often heartbreaking skin condition that continues in spite of sufferers' fighting—and spending—to resolve it.

Indeed, according to J. E. Barnes, "Female adults are seeking treatments much more often than in the past, raising sales of everything from body washes to birth control pills on their quest for clear skin."[1] As a result, Barnes pointed out, "skin care and drug companies have seized on—and perhaps exploited—the trend, bombarding women with ads that play on the insecurities of young adults with less-than-perfect skin and explicitly discuss new, more effective treatments."[2] That is why sales of anti-acne medications in supermarkets and drugstores were almost $400 million in 2001, according to A. C. Nielsen, the store auditing specialists. Also, sales of acne prescriptions grew around 20 percent between 1998 and 2001. And this prescription figure doesn't even include the large number of birth control prescriptions written partly or wholly to resolve acne. For example, sale of Ortho TriCyclen, a low-dosage birth control pill, rose from $225 million in 1998 to over $500 million in 2001 since its owners, Johnson and Johnson, started advertising that it was an effective acne cure.[3]

ELIMINATING ACNE IS VITAL

Good-looking, healthy skin is important for everyone. We all know what a problem acne can be for young people.

"People who don't have acne don't know the pain," wrote 15-year-old Jeremy on the Internet. "I just wanted to give up living. . . . That's how bad it was."[4]

But not only teenagers suffer. So do adults. For example, executives are often judged at least to some extent by the appearance of their skin. As John Challenger, CEO of Challenger, Gray and Christmas, a leading outplacement firm, put it, "If someone comes in and seems to be breaking out all over in acne, that can cause the other person discomfort. And that could undermine the interview."[5]

A female who is a successful sales executive confided, "My next promotion may be in jeopardy if my skin looks real bad. It's not fair. But I can't really blame my boss. He's right. I'd be less effective making a sales pitch to some senior guy if my face is covered in spots."

"It's like Neutrogena says in their ads," another woman told us. "Acne stands out more in an adult."

The fact is that acne, if it is left untreated—or is ineffectively treated—can be a real curse for people young and old.

IT MAY BE GETTING WORSE

There is some evidence that the incidence of acne, at least in adult women, is on the rise. Two studies conducted by the English University of Leeds in 1979 and 1996, show that there was an increase in the incidence of acne in women from 35 percent to 54 percent.[6,7] No one knows exactly why this is, or whether it would apply to women in America, but many observers believe it would.

Theories abound as to why adult female acne is rising. One of the most plausible is that the increase is the result of the greater stress women face as they advance to increasingly senior career positions. Moreover, acne in women is more visible than it used to be. For one thing, women working outside the home, unlike homemakers, cannot afford to stay out of sight when their acne flares up. For another, since heavy makeup is well out of fashion, gone are the days when women could cover blemishes by slathering on foundation. "Nowadays you have to cure the problem, not cover it up," one woman explained when Brenda Adderly interviewed her.

DON'T BELIEVE THE NAYSAYERS

In a 1998 paper, three eminent UCLA physicians—Richard Usatine, director of predoctoral education; Martin Quan, residency director of the Family Medicine Program; and Richard Strick, clinical professor of dermatology and medicine—correctly stated that acne "can be painful both physically and psychologically. Inflamed lesions can hurt, and acne breakouts can result in low self-esteem, loss of self-confidence, social isolation, and even depression." Unfortunately, they also stated that "though acne is not generally cured, treatment can reduce the severity and frequency of outbreaks, lessen discomfort from inflamed lesions, improve appearance, and prevent or minimize scarring, thereby averting or ameliorating potentially serious adverse psychosocial effects."[7]

Whether or not one calls the protocol we have outlined in this book a "cure" is a matter of semantics. But we believe that when physicians write that the problem cannot be completely resolved and can only be "reduced in severity and frequency," this clinical conservatism is likely to mislead patients. In everyday parlance, effectively eliminating the symptoms of acne in 95 percent of all cases by the simple protocol we have outlined—and eliminating the other 5 percent by additional medical means—constitutes a cure. To imply that the best that can be done is to "lessen discomfort," "minimize scarring," and "reduce the severity" of acne is to allow medical conservatism to transmute into medical inaccuracy.

Pessimistic thinking by the finest professionals in the field inevitably infects all thinking on the subject of acne. When you look up acne and its treatment on the Internet, you find pages of "support" groups, long-term acne "programs," "living with acne" Web sites, and "controlling acne" advisors. To cite just one example, Facefacts by Roche (one of the world's largest pharmaceutical companies) offers "a progressive coaching program designed to work with you through your acne treatment."[8] This and other help and advisory groups operate on the tacit assumption that acne is incurable, something you have to live with, one of life's inevitable slings and arrows.

Moreover, people who suffer from acne are offered "cures" galore. But they don't work. No doubt, then, the circumstantial evidence suggests that the experts are correct when they state—or at least strongly imply—that acne cannot be cured, only controlled, and that not very well. No wonder that acne sufferers assume a victim mentality.

But as prescribed in chapter 4, apply salicylic acid to your skin. Then use glycolic acid. Follow that by benzoyl peroxide applied to cooled skin—and, within no more than 6 weeks, your acne will be eliminated. Gone. And good riddance!

Will it return? If you follow our protocol for good skin care, probably not. If you also lower your stress, take the recommended supplements, and stay healthy, almost certainly not. And if it does return, it will be very much milder, and very quickly resolved.

So don't believe the naysayers.

THE ULTIMATE REWARD

"Rose cheeked Laura," the poet Thomas Campion called his love, and in 1617 he wrote of her:

There is a garden in her face

Where roses and white lilies grow;

A heavenly paradise is that place

Wherein all pleasant fruits do flow.

Shakespeare extolled the beauty of his love's face in many an immortal sonnet, once describing her complexion as "smooth as . . . alabaster." Christopher Marlowe had Faust say of Helen of Troy:

Oh, thou art fairer than the evening air

Clad in the beauty of a thousand stars.

And Emerson said, "If eyes were made for seeing, then Beauty is its own excuse for being."

We have a long tradition of loving, admiring, exalting, adoring beauty. We adulate film stars—from Greta Garbo to Marilyn Monroe to Julia Roberts—for their beauty. But no beauty, not of the 16th century nor of today, would be so lovely if her face were covered with zits.

Nor, for that matter, would the great masculine seducers—from Adonis to Don Juan, from Valentino to Brad Pitt—be as desirable were their faces marred with acne pimples and pustules and pits.

Clearly, clearly, to rise to those heights—or, for that matter, to attract that charming boy or girl next door—you need to beat back the skin disease that is acne.

And now you can.

So let us end where we started. . . .

Follow the protocol outlined in this book and, in 95 cases out of 100, within no more than 6 weeks (and often less), you will be acne-free. (In the other five cases, the acne will be much less severe, but it may take a few more steps to eradicate it completely.) Then, once you have completed the Acne Cure program and your face is unblemished, by following our simple skin care program, you can be sure it will stay that way. In fact, chances are that your skin will continue to improve—and then stay at its best for many years to come.

And the result for you?

Why, nothing much . . . just that you will look great and feel as good as you look. From the inside out, and on the outside for all the world to see, you will positively glow!

ENDNOTES

CHAPTER 1

1. The Associated Press, "U.S. Youth Burning to Get Suntans,"*International Herald Tribune*, June 3, 2002.

2. Vedantam, S., "In a Study of the Brain, Special Nerves Registered the Emotional Context of a Pleasurable Touch,"*The Washington Post*, July 29, 2002, A2.

CHAPTER 2

1. David J. Leffell, M.D., *Total Skin* (New York: Hyperion, 2000), 330.

2. Kelly Bartlett, "Pubescent Lament," Creative Writing for Teens www.teen-writing.about.com; published January 1998.

3.The Acne Support Group, P.O. Box 9, Newquay, Cornwall TR9 6WG, England. Telephone: 011-44-0870-870-2263.

4. Anthony C. Chu, M.D., and Anne Lovell, *The Good Skin Doctor* (London: Thorsons, 1999), vii.

5. Ibid, 80.

6. Ibid, 79.

7. Acne Net, American Academy of Dermatology, www.skincarephysicians.com/acnenet/socimpct.html; accessed August 2002.

8. Ibid.

CHAPTER 4

1. Nicholas Perricone, M.D., *The Wrinkle Cure* (New York: Warner, 2000), 98.

2. Ibid, 94.

3. Anthony C. Chu and Anne Lovell, *The Good Skin Doctor* (London: Thorsons, 1999), 96.

CHAPTER 5

1. E. Zander and S. Weisman, "Treatment of Acne Vulgaris with Salicylic Acid Pads," *Clinical Therapies*, vol. 14, no. 2, March–April 1992, 247–53.

2. B. A. Johnson and J. R. Nunley, "Topical Therapy for Acne Vulgaris. How Do You Choose the Best Drug for Each Patient?" *Postgraduate Medicine*, vol. 107, no. 3, March 2000, 69–70, 73–76, 79–80.

3. Z. Fendrich et al., "Effective and Safe Pharmacotherapy of Acne Vulgaris and

Treatment of Sun-Damaged Skin," *Czech and Slovak Pharmacy*, vol. 49, no. 2, March 2000, 62–67.

4. A. R. Shalita, "Treatment of Mild and Moderate Acne Vulgaris with Salicylic Acid in an Alcohol–Detergent Vehicle," *Cutis*, vol. 28, no. 5, November 1981, 556–58, 561.

5. A.R. Shalita, "Comparison of salicylic acid cleanser and a benzoyl peroxide wash in the treatment of acne vulgaris," *Clinical Therapies*, vol.11, no. 2, March-April 1989, 264–67.

6. P. E. Grimes, "The Safety and Efficacy of Salicylic Acid and Chemical Peels in Darker Racial-Ethnic Groups," *Dermatologic Surgery*, vol. 25, no. 1, January 1999, 18–22.

7. W. P. Smith, "Comparative Effectiveness of A-Hydroxy Acids on Skin Properties," *International Journal of Cosmetic Science*, vol. 18, 1996, 75–83.

8. R. C. Tung et al., "Alpha-Hydroxy Acid–Based Cosmetic Procedures: Guidelines for Patient Management," *American Journal of Clinical Dermatology*, vol. 1, no. 2, March–April 2000, 81–88.

9. E. J. Van Scott et al., "Hyperkeratinization, Corneocyte Cohesion, and Alpha Hydroxyl Acids," *Journal of the American Academy of Dermatology*, vol. 11, no. 5, part 1, August 2001, 867–79.

10. L. Atzori et al., "Glycolic Acid Peeling in the Treatment of Acne," *Journal of European Academy of Dermatology*, vol. 12, no. 2, March 1999, 119–22.

11. M. C. Spellman and S. H. Pincus, "Efficacy and Safety of Azelaic Acid and Glycolic Acid Combination Therapy Compared with Tretinoin Therapy for Acne," *Clinical Therapies*, vol. 20, no. 4, July 1998, 711–21.

12. C. M. Wang et al., "The Effect of Glycolic Acid on the Treatment of Acne in Asian Skin," *Dermatological Surgery*, vol. 23, no. 1, January 1997, 23–29.

13. M. Kharfi et al., " 'Comparative Study of the Efficacy and Tolerance of 12% Glycolic Acid Cream and 0.05% Retinoic Acid Cream for Polymorphic Acne," *Tunis Medicine*, vol. 79, nos. 6–7, June–July 2001, 374–77.

14. Z. Erbagci and C. Akcali, "Biweekly Serial Glycolic Acid Peels vs. Long-Term Daily Use of Topical Low-Strength Glycolic Acid in the Treatment of Atrophic Acne Scars," *International Journal of Dermatology*, vol. 39, no. 10, October 2000, 789–94.

15. Wang et al., "The Effect of Glycolic Acid on the Treatment of Acne in Asian Skin," 23–29.

16. N. V. Perricone and J. C. DiNardo, "Photoprotective and Anti-Inflammatory Effects of Topical Glycolic Acid," *Dermatologic Surgery*, vol. 22, no. 5, May 1996, 435–37.

17. J. C. DiNardo et al., "Clinical and Histological Effects of Glycolic Acid at Different Concentrations and pH Levels," *Dermatologic Surgery*, vol. 22, no. 5, May 1996, 421–24.

18. Ibid.

19. P. K. Thibault et al., "A Double-Blind Randomized Clinical Trial on the Effectiveness of a Daily Glycolic Acid 5% Formulation in the Treatment of Photoaging," *Dermatologic Surgery*, vol. 24, no. 5, May 1998, 573–78.

20. A. M. Kligman, *Acne and Rosacea*, second ed., (Heidelberg: Springer Verlag, 1993), 599–600.

21. N. Hjorth, "Traditional Topical Treatment of Acne," *Acta Derm Veneresol Supp* (Stockholm), Sup 89, 1980, 53–56.

22. J. J. Leyden et al., "Comparison of the Efficacy and Safety of a Combination of Topical Gel Formulation of Benzoyl Peroxide and Clindamycin with Benzoyl Peroxide, Clindamycin and Vehicle Gel in the Treatments of Acne Vulgaris," *American Journal of Clinical Dermatology*, vol. 2, no. 1, 2001, 33–39.

23. J. J. Leyden et al., "The Efficacy and Safety of a Combination Benzoyl Peroxide/Clindamycin Topical Gel Compared with Benzoyl Peroxide Alone and a Benzoyl Peroxide/Erythromycin Combination Product," *Journal of Cutaneous Medicine and Surgery*, vol. 5, no. 1, January–February 2001, 37–42.

24. J. J. Leyden and S. Levy, "The Development of Antibiotic Resistance in Propionibacterium Acnes," *Cutis*, vol. 67, 2 suppl., February 2001, 21–24.

25. A. M. Kligman, "Acne Vulgaris: Tricks and Treatments. Part II: The Benzoyl Peroxide Saga," *Cutis*, vol. 56, no. 2, November 1995, 260.

26. V. B. Patel et al., "Preparation and Comparative Clinical Evaluation of Liposomal Gel of Benzoyl Peroxide for Acne," *Drug Development Ind Pharm*, vol. 27, no. 8, September 2001, 863–69.

27. G. Valacci et al., "Effect of Benzoyl Peroxide on Antioxidant Status. NF-kappaB Activity and Interleukin-1 Alpha Gene Expression in Human Keratinocytes," *Toxicology*, vol. 165, nos. 2–3, August 2001, 225–34.

CHAPTER 6

1. Nicholas Perricone, M.D., *The Wrinkle Cure* (New York: Warner, 2000), 1.

2. David J. Leffell, M.D., *Total Skin* (New York: Hyperion, 2000), 61.

3. M. P. Lupo, "Antioxidants and Vitamins in Cosmetics," *Clinics in Dermatology*, vol. 19, no. 4, July–August 2000, 467–73.

4. Jurgen Fuchs, Lester Packer, Guido Zimmer, Arno B. Zimmer, Editors *Lipoic Acid in Health and Disease* (New York: Marcel Dekker, 1997), 43.

5. G. J. Fisher et al., "Pathophysiology of Premature Skin Aging Induced by Ultraviolet Light," *New England Journal of Medicine*, no. 337, November 13, 1997, 1419–29.

6. L. H. Kligman et al., "Topical Retinoic Acid Enhances the Repair of Ultravi-

olet Damaged Dermal Connective Tissue," *Connective Tissue Research*, vol.12, –no. 2, 1984, 139–50.

7. A. M. Kligman et al., "Topical Tretinoin for Photoaged Skin," *Journal of the American Academy of Dermatology*, vol. 15, no. 4, part 2, October 1986, 838–59.

8. J. S. Weiss et al., "Topical Tretinoin (Retinoic Acid) Improves Photoaged Skin. A double-blind vehicle-controlled study," *Journal of the American Medical Association*, no. 259, vol. 4, January 1988, 527–32.

9. F. A. Schwartz et al., "Topical All-Trans-Retinoic Acid Stimulates Collagen Synthesis in Vivo," *Journal of Investigative Dermatology*, vol. 96, no. 6, 1991, 975–78.

10. E. S. Rafal et al., "Topical Tretinoin (Retinoic Acid) Treatment for Liver Spots Associated with Photodamage," *New England Journal of Medicine*, vol. 326, no. 6, 1992, 368–74.

11. R. Kotrajaras and A. M. Kligman, "The Effect of Topical Tretinoin on Photodamaged Facial Skin: The Thai Experience," *British Journal of Dermatology*, vol. 129, no. 3, September 1993, 302–309.

12. B. A. Gilchrest, "A Review of Skin Ageing and Its Medical Therapy," *British Journal of Dermatology*, vol. 135, no. 6, December 1996, 867–75.

13. C. E. M. Griffiths, "Nicotinamide 4% Gel for the Treatment of Inflammatory Acne Vulgaris," *Journal of Dermatology Treatment*, vol. 6, 1995, S8–10.

14. R. E. Fitzpatrick and E. F. Rostan, "Double-Blind, Half-Face Study Comparing Topical Vitamin C and Vehicle for Rejuvenation of Photodamage," *Dermatology Surgery*, vol. 28, no. 3, March 2002, 231–36.

15. L. S. Baumann and J. Spencer, "The Effects of Topical Vitamin E on the Cosmetic Appearance of Scars," *Dermatology Surgery*, vol. 25, no. 4, April 1999, 311–15.

16. Lupo, "Antioxidants and Vitamins in Cosmetics," 467-73.

17. G. Michaelsson et al., "A Double-Blind Study of the Effect of Zinc and Oxytetracycline in Acne Vulgaris," *British Journal of Dermatology*, vol. 97, no. 5, November 1977, 561–66.

18. G. Michaelsson et al., "Effects of Oral Zinc and Vitamin A in Acne," *Archives of Dermatology*, vol. 113, no.1, 1977, 31.

19. G. Michaelsson and L. E. Edquist, *Acta Derm Venereol*, vol. 64, no.1, 1984, 14.

CHAPTER 7

1. S. Okie, "Diet Rich in Vitamins C, E May Pare Alzheimer's Risk," *Washington Post*, June 26, 2002, section A.

2. M. J. Engelhart et al., "Dietary Intake of Antioxidants and Risk of Alzheimer's

Disease," *Journal of the American Medical Association*, vol. 278, no. 24, June 26, 2002, 3223–29.

3. Nicholas Perricone, M.D., *The Wrinkle Cure* (New York: Warner, 2000), 131.

CHAPTER 9

1. Neil Persadsingh, *Acne in Black Women,* (Jamaica, West Indies: Self-published, 1998), 1.

2. Ibid, 25.

3. J. E. Fulton, "Acne: Its Causes and Treatments," *Brunei International Medical Journal*, vol.1, 1999, 45–58.

CHAPTER 10

1. Martha Davis, Ph.D., Elizabeth Robbins Eshelman, M.S.W., Matthew McKay, Ph.D., *The Relaxation and Stress Reduction Workbook* (Oakland, California: New Harbinger, 2000), 10.

2. Ibid, 9.

3. C. Saindon, "Can't Sleep? 15 Tips You Can Try," www.selfhelpmagazine.com/articles/trauma/trsleep.html; accessed July 2002.

CHAPTER 11

1. Carol Turkington and Jeffrey Dover, M.D., *Skin Deep* (New York: Facts on File, 1998), 4.

CHAPTER 13

1. Peter Engel and Merrit Malloy, *Old Wives' Tales: The Truth about Everyday Myths* (New York: St. Martin's, 1993), 15.

2. Carol Turkington and Jeffrey Dover, M.D., *Skin Deep* (New York: Facts on File, 1998), 6.

3. J. E. Fulton, "Acne: Its Causes and Treatments," *Brunei International Medical Journal*, vol. 1, 1991, 45–58.

4. Myriam Zaoui and Eric Malka, *The Art of Shaving* (New York: Clarkson/Potter, 2002), 33.

CHAPTER 14

1. J. E. Barnes, "Acne: No Longer Just a Market for Teenagers," *New York Times*, April 27, 2001, Business section.

2. Ibid.

3. Ibid.

4. Jeremy, "Pubescent Lament," Creative Writing for Teens www.teenwriting. about.com; accessed January 1998.

5. J. E. Barnes, "Acne: No Longer Just a Market for Teenagers," *New York Times*, April 27, 2001, Business section.

6. W. J. Cunliffe and D. J. Gould, "Prevalence of Facial Acne Vulgaris in Late Adolescence and in Adults," *British Medical Journal,* vol. 1, 1979, 1109–10.

7. V. Goulden et al., "Post-Adolescent Acne: A Review of Clinical Features," *British Journal of Dermatology,* vol. 136, 1997, 66–70.

8. R. P. Usatine et al., "Acne Vulgaris: A Treatment Update," *Hospital Practice*, vol. 23, no. 3, February 1998, 111.

9. F.A.C.E. Program, www.facefacts.com/program_home.asp; accessed July 2002.

INDEX

Underscored page references indicate boxed text.

Foods
  effect of cooking, 98
  misconceptions about, 188–91
  processed vs. nonprocessed, 16
  rich in
    B vitamins, 89, 103
    calcium, 108
    chromium, 109
    magnesium, 108
    selenium, 110
    vitamin C, 100
    vitamin E, 104
    zinc, 110
France, eating habits in, 99
Free radicals, 14–16, 53

Gamma tocopherol, 104
Genetics, 184, 197
Glutathione peroxidase, 109
Glycation, of collagen, 102
Glycolic acid, 53–54, 84
  on Black skin, 67, 135
  characteristics of, 55–56
  for chemical peels, 178, 179
  instructions for using, 56, 95
  research on effectiveness of, 66–69
  using cold with, 59
Gly Derm, 56
Good Skin Doctor, The, 57
Granulation tissue, 173, 174
Grease, airborne, 30–31
Grisefulvin, 194

Hair, Black
  effect of glycolic acid on, 135
  products for, 133–34, 160
Hair, body
  evolution of, 21–22
  waxing, 193
Hair, facial. See also Shaving
  thickness of, 187–88
  unshaved, 117–18
Hair follicles. See also Pilosebaceous
        follicles; Pores
  plugged, 37–39
  role in acne of, 19
Hair products, 160–61
  for Black hair, 133–34, 160
Hairs, ingrown. See Ingrown hairs
Halothane, 164
Heredity, role in acne of, 184, 197

High potency E (HPE), 92–93, 104.
      See also Tocotrienol
Hispanic skin, 132, 133, 134, 138
Homocysteine levels, 103
Hormones
  in men, 185
  in teenagers, 187
  in women, 40, 164, 185
HPE. See High potency E
Humectants, 89
Hydroquinine cream, 178
Hydroxyl radicals, 53
Hygiene, in history, 22. See also
      Skin, cleansing
Hyperkeratinization, 67
Hyperpigmentation, 178
Hypertrophic scarring, 174

Ice pick scars, 25, 173, 180
  removing, 181
Imaginary acne, 161
Immune system, 103
  effect on
    of stress, 146
    of vitamin C, 89, 100–101
    of zinc, 110
Infant acne, 165, 184–85
Infections. see also Bacteria;
        Propionibacterium
  cysts formed by, 42
  secondary, 57, 195
  skin's self-protection from, 5–6
  spreading of, 184
Inflammation, 27, 57
  around ingrown hairs, 119–20
  in Black skin, 132
  reducing, 51
    with alpha lipoic acid, 102
    with cold, 58–59, 60–61, 64
    with salicylic acid, 53
    with vitamin C, 91
  role in scarring of, 172–73
Infrared light, 78
  in laser dermabrasion, 180
Ingrown hairs, 118–23
  acne vs., 120–21
  in Black men, 132
  eliminating, 121–23
  reasons for, 119
Insecticides, exposure to, 165–66
Insulation, subcutaneous layer as, 20

212